Honoring The Calling

Escaping the Abyss

Richard J. Stephens Jr., MA

Ozark Publishing

Contents

"We have two wolves inside each of us, one honorable, one evil. The winner is the one we choose to feed."

Dr. Larue

Chapter One

Acknowledgment

As we travel this journey called life, I have found that it is impossible to traverse the ground, rough or level, without the helpful guidance of those we hold most dear. This continuation of my journey does not fail to encompass that fact and wouldn't have been possible without the continued support and guidance from my beautiful wife Leona. Leona's constant reminders, encouragement, and grounding paved the way for me to expound on the original Calling book, exploring the safeguards we often implement once we recognize that our lives are becoming affected by stress, trauma, and darkness. Through her I have found inspiration and a sincere resolve to continue the fight.

Chapter Two

Introduction

To truly honor the chosen calling of being a peace officer, in these modern times, one must exhibit a willingness to recognize and confront the unpleasant segments of the mission. A thing we value, revere, and hold in high regard, the police officers calling not only includes our service to our communities and all of those falling under its blanket but likewise ourselves. Recognizing and taking active steps towards repairing the damage caused to us personally, from a lifetime of service and our subsequent engaging in active measures to ensure we do not sink is not unlike the ship repairman of old, recognizing the danger of a hole in the ship, seeking out remedies and repairing the damage to continue the journey.

Recognizing that the byproduct of life as a law enforcement official, veteran, or truly anyone in the service of others involves trauma, some resolved and some unresolved, one must be prepared to confront the proverbial demons to experience sustained wellness. Not unlike me personally, many who have been honored to have worn or continue to wear a badge, following the noble calling of service, easily fall into a chasm of darkness which affects not only their own personal health but likewise their actions and behaviors as they move past the events they experience.

Throughout the original *The Calling* book, we explored the cause-and-effect realities of who public servants are and why they do the things they do. Although many choose the career for reasons relating to service, notoriety, or out of obligation, no central reasoning of why they choose to serve is apparent. Where one may enter the field because generations of his family have served before him, others begin because of a deep yearning to simply help their community.

Some begin their service because of things they have observed in person. Some start because of the intense desire to look cool, drive fast, and shoot guns. Although differing in reasoning for service one thing is consistent among those serving. It is assured that all those serving will be bombarded with trauma from the moment they arrive for their first shift until the day they choose to hang up the leather and call it quits.

Believing that retiring from the field will become the catalyst for a healthy recovery, many quickly realize the concept that simply riding off into the sunset will mend their proverbial wounds, allowing them a sense of satisfaction and contentment for the life of service they lived, quickly learn is in error. This error stems from their struggle with not only the demons of years of experiences, mislabeled, and neglected, but new trauma of exclusion from the very brotherhood they held so high for the duration of their careers.

Getting to the point of recognizing the need for addressing unresolved trauma and seeking help is a slippery slope for many within the law enforcement field. Being providers, warriors, and often superheroes in the minds of many, causes the mass majority of those serving to fail to recognize the need for addressing their emotional health. Coupled with the inability to recognize the need, many within the realm simply consider the baggage associated with their chosen calling to be a part of the norm and objectifying it would in a sense render them weaker on some level. Although this mentality couldn't be farther from the truth, in all reality, it's valid to many.

Fostering relationships and striving to shift the proverbial "norm" from that of disbelief and hesitation, into recognition and acceptance is a never-ending battle for all of those who truly care enough about these professionals and their ongoing health. Throughout this continuation of the Calling series, we will explore the wide array of concepts and actionable items which have been placed into motion to offset the damage caused by the field itself. Whether an officer chooses conventional means of assistance such as therapy or peer related counseling, or more non-conventional means similar to exploring the faith factor, holistic remedies, or other approaches designed to enhance one's health, the end goal remains.

Exploring each possible remedy can be beneficial if the officer himself or herself takes ownership and can truly see the value therein. The crux for all practical accounts is determining exactly how to meet the needs of each individual officer, building upon their commitment and resiliency. Meeting those needs includes taking the time necessary to lessen any stigmas related to seeking assistance and building upon the necessity of action rather than inaction. Simply said, we must make the fact that the trauma associated with their chosen career is real and must be addressed. Likewise, addressing the issues at hand must be accompanied by a flexible and innovative series of remedies which will meet the needs of each individual officer. A one size fits all approach is pointless on every level. Although some may disagree, this fact is simply reality.

Continuing our walk in the shoes of those serving our communities, we must recognize that for some, the traditional concepts of formal therapy and behavioral health services simply are not an option. Not that they couldn't or wouldn't be beneficial, rather because some officers refuse to accept the possibility of engaging on that level due to highly personal reasons and yes, the perceived stigma associated with the need for assistance under the guise of professional therapy.

In a sense, as we begin this continuation of our journey, we find ourselves in an abyss of sorts. As defined by Webster's Dictionary (2021), "a deep seemingly bottomless chasm" the result of a lifetime of service, witnessing the depravity of mankind and the darkness of our world around us. The key is recognizing and then placing into motion a series of strategies designed to conquer this latest mission, ensuring wellness and resiliency for the very servants we owe so much to. Here we will explore and overcome.

Chapter Three

The Pack / Leader Mentality

"I woke up one morning thinking about wolves and realized that wolf packs function as families. Everyone has a role, and if you act within the parameters of your role, the whole pack succeeds, and when that falls apart, so does the pack"

~ Jodi Picoult

As a young man, I remember watching a movie which depicted a small pack of wolves in the wild. Becoming enthralled with what I was seeing, my interest was piqued, and I began researching every aspect of this majestic yet seemingly honorable beast. Desiring to learn more about the species, I seldom missed any opportunity to read, watch, or even visit anything associated with wolves as they became available. Over time, the mere glimpse of a wolf, regardless of if it was in a printed picture or on the television screen caused a calming within my inner most being.

What caused this interest? I have no idea. The topic wasn't something which my family instilled upon me. Nor was I a member of any rescue or interest groups. My interest was purely self-driven, seemingly the answer to something I was pinning up deep inside of me. Working in the mountains of Colorado provided me with the perfect opportunity to not only engage my interest in wolves but also for the first time, view one in person. I remember learning of a local citizen who had applied for and received the necessary governmental approval to create a wolf refuge. Upon tracking the citizen down, I decided that, while patrolling one day, I would make a visit in hopes of obtaining information and creating a learning experience for me.

As I entered the property, my eyes immediately were drawn to the silver and white coat of a large wolf standing along the ridgeline. I recall being seated in silence as I looked somberly at this majestic creature for the first time. Its size astonished me. What I had envisioned as a normal-sized dog in all reality was nothing further from the truth. Its tall lengthy stature stood out as I watched the single wolf stand, overlooking his fellow pack members, seemingly standing guard, prepared to ward off any attack from those intending to cause the pack harm. The excitement of the moment, finally seeing one in the wild, per se, seemed to fill my final need for research at that point.

Thinking back on my love for the wolf as a species, I can now understand where my desire to learn stemmed from. Deep inside me, I as with many men and women who choose to enter the realm of law enforcement possess many characteristics of the wolf and the pack in general. Although many others have penned negative descriptions of the "wolf pack concept", I have long believed that one particular attribute often found in wolf packs reigns supreme. Like a pack, the inner yearning to provide and protect is an essential, nonvisible characteristic which is deeply engrained within not only me, but I would suffice to say almost every successful law enforcement officer. As with the wolf, those wearing the badge truly encompass the attribute of caring about very little other than providing and protecting, even when they may not recognize it.

As officers carry out their routine duties of serving their communities, everything they do revolves around ensuring that those within their communities remain safe and are provided with all the necessary resources to sustain life and succeed. The wolf mentality encompasses more than simply those people our law enforcement men and women serve but in fact revolves more stringently around the brotherhood they create with those serving alongside them, not only within their individual agency but with other agencies, officers, and in fact anyone wearing the badge.

The individual law enforcement officer, unknowingly in some cases, carries out his or her duties on a day-to-day basis with one specific goal in mind. That goal being ensuring the protection and welfare of his or her pack through providing them with the essential items needed to survive. This aspect of police culture is what makes it so difficult for others within our community, many times with similar goals, to break down the proverbial safety walls within the law enforcement community and be trusted.

I remember, shortly after beginning my work as a Community Behavioral Health Liaison in the state of Missouri, listening to a fellow behavioral health professional describe how he had come under a moderate amount of scrutiny because he was unable to gain the acceptance of a certain counties law enforcement and court personnel. As my co-worker spoke, he described that he traveled along with his supervisor and tried aimlessly to break down the barriers to communication and gain cooperation from the agency. The resource this gentle man and his team were offering was a no brainer, for the most part, and without a doubt would greatly benefit any organization or community.

Following pitching their product per se, the team returned to their vehicle and simply looked at each other, discussing how difficult that interaction had been and how they felt at a loss over how to break down the barriers and show the law enforcement officials in that area their intent was pure and reasonable. As I listened intently, I shifted in my chair and couldn't resist providing my friend with the answer he was seeking. "Do you want to know why?" I said, with a slight grin on my face. As my question caught his attention, he turned, and I began describing why he struggled to engage those within law enforcement.

My friend's inability to connect with that county official wasn't because he didn't give it his all. Similarly, it wasn't because he was uneducated or the product, he was offering was sub-par or lacked substantial benefit to the officials. It was merely because he was a man, outside the pack, trying to gain admittance. Being driven to protect and provide has left many, and I would suffice to say, if not all of those within the law enforcement community to trust nothing that comes from outside the pack, regardless of how pristine the packaging is or how grand it looks. This lack of trust reveals itself on multiple levels but in the end, it exists and is a powerful force.

Law enforcement officials and all of those associated with the field fall into a preservation mentality after working within the field for a relatively short time. You quickly learn that you can only truly rely on your brothers and sisters for support because they are the only ones who truly understand what you are going through. The onslaught of false media perspectives, on screen depictions and ongoing anti- police narratives fuel the thought that it is only within the confines of the pack that trust can be found. This creates a deep burning deep inside each officer where their view of anyone outside the field is adversely affected.

When someone outside the law enforcement community attempts to break down the protective walls and gain admittance, the law enforcement mind, although cordial, remains skeptical, waiting for the shoe to drop and the newly admitted member to attack. In many cases this couldn't be furthest from the truth, but it remains the reality of interaction. As described by Steven Cox, (2019) "The police subculture, or blue fraternity or brotherhood, consists of the informal rules and regulations, tactics, and folklore passed on from one generation of police officers to another. It's both the result and cause of police isolation from the larger society". In the mind of the normal everyday police officer, Trooper, and Sheriff's Deputy, anyone outside the pack or group, cannot fully be trusted to act in the best interest of the pack, hence remaining professional, welcoming, and kind is essential but following up and engaging the outsider is pointless and potentially wrought with danger.

This, in a nutshell, was what had happened to my friend. He arrived telling tales of how he was there to help and make the lives of law enforcement officers throughout the area much easier, as they went about their jobs of serving the public. But in the mind of those officers, the question of whether he could be trusted remained unanswered, hence they smiled and placed the info in the "special file" most likely never to be considered again. The normal need of law enforcement officers to protect not only himself or herself as well as the health and wellness of his fellow brothers and sisters rises to an entirely enhanced level when one adds the police administrator to the mix.

Routinely stemming from a lengthy bout within the police culture, the modern police administrator possesses the same shared beliefs and concepts which are prevalent within the subculture. As a product of the leadership position itself, I would love to be able to say that police administrators miraculously do not have to face the same leadership stressors civilian and military leaders do but claiming that would be in error. In spite of an extremely protective brotherhood where "I have your back" is a common theme, police administrators are seemingly forgotten to an extent. The jargon of loudly supporting and silent dissent seems to many times be lost in the process where police administrators are concerned. The modern police leader faces the same, second guessing, silent and many times vocal dissent in the deep corners of the patrol room that other modern leaders do. This factor does little more than add to the stress felt by police administrators.

Regardless of the aforementioned detractors, the modern police leader remains steadfast on his ultimate goal. The one thing that he or she has learned from years of service to not only his community but likewise to his brothers and sisters, trust no one, especially those outside. Having this deeply instilled belief causes those within the administrative and leadership realm of law enforcement to question, many times silently, and change or shift in methodology as it relates not only to himself but to his pack or people. Hence, he becomes fiercely protective of his pack and becomes ever watchful for anything attempting to cause harm.

As we discuss the pack and protector mentality, I would like to take a moment and explain something extremely important. Some may read these words and disagree or question the methodology and conclusions drawn. That is completely acceptable, but I would hope that you will broaden your perspective because as outlandish as it may appear, it's a reality. My worldview stems from an extensive education and experience lasting over thirty years in the field, daily interacting with my brothers and sisters bearing the badge. The thought of trust and alienation of outsiders is not an open concept. When dealing with our law enforcement officials we are dealing with, in my opinion, some of the most educated, tactically sound, and brilliant individuals who have ever walked the earth. They are men and women who have fine-tuned the art of camouflage and learn to skillfully gain cooperation from the most trying individuals and circumstances. In saying this, one must understand that this lack of trust is a silent attribute and seldom voiced or visualized. Rather, it remains in the mind of the officer and is exposed many times through inaction.

The concepts of law enforcement officers and leaders being fiercely protective of their packs and desiring to merely safeguard and provide for their own has some unfortunate results in some instances. Having this mentality many times causes a breakdown in modernization and moving forward with innovative concepts. Throughout this journey we will address one such breakdown, the lack of those within the police sub-culture to fully accept when new concepts surrounding wellness and resiliency are necessary. Fully grasping the need for potential shifts in the manner we conduct business is a tough one for many within law enforcement. Change requires a full vetting of content and associations to ensure the protection of the pack. Understanding why we hesitate is essential.

Chapter Summary and Key Takeaways

· Like the wolf pack, wolf culture, law enforcement officers have a deeply seated desire and need to protect and provide for their fellow officers. This desire often facilitates a lack of trust for anyone outside their pack.

· The police subculture fosters secrecy. This attribute can cause hesitation to fully grasp modern concepts of health and wellness needs.

· Those filling leadership roles within the modern law enforcement organization likewise shift their beliefs to that of protector and provider, feeling an obligation to not only protect themselves but the entirety of the pack in the face of leadership stressors.

Chapter Four

Police Culture Creates Hesitation

"Make up your mind to act decidedly and take the consequences. No good is ever done in the world by hesitation."

~Thomas Huxley

A s my family struggled with the ailing health of one of our beloved pets, I sprang into action. Taking charge during difficult times had become the norm for me. As my mother had penned it many years prior, I simply kicked into "cop mode" and rid myself of any and all emotion, striving to remedy the situation and keep everyone near me safe and calm. Cop mode, as mom described, was simply when I took charge and took every burden upon myself, stone faced, and acted in the best interest of the family. An intriguing behavioral characteristic, in its most simplistic form, where I simply pushed everything to the side and acted out of a pure, unabridged absence of emotion, concerned only about others. On this night, our aging toy poodle, Isie, my wife's pride, and joy, had drawn near to her last days. She had been experiencing bouts of passing out due to heart complications and many times had to be revived because we simply couldn't bear saying goodbye.

As she entered into another seizure like incident, I quickly revived her and as she sat in her human mother's lap, striving to regain her footing and balance, I quietly sat on the couch adjacent to my wife. As our daughters gathered around their mother and our baby, Isie, I somberly watched and silently prayed that God give Leona, my wife, and the girls strength to hold up under the loss we would surely soon experience. Thinking little about anything other than my girls and ultimately maintaining my composure, considering this little furry baby had been a part of my life for the past twelve years, I sat in silence.

Within moments my youngest child, nine-year-old Riyann, walked over to where I sat, placing her hand on my shoulder, saying "it's ok to cry daddy." Doing my best to maintain my stern dad, protector vibe, I smiled and simply responded that I knew, and I appreciated her. She then patted my shoulder, gently, and added "daddy, you are not a cop any more...you can let your emotions out and cry... it's ok now." This little girl went on to say, "It's ok to feel and let your emotions show daddy." Without hesitation this little child not only recognized the existence of hesitation present in the lives of her dear old dad and all those serving within the field of law enforcement, but she also did her best to encourage me to recognize the pain and allow my emotions to flow. Assuring her that I understood and that I was alright, although momentarily finding it difficult, I rapidly assumed my fallback position of straight-faced compliance to the order of man and simply placed what I was feeling inside to the back burner and rekindled my need to be strong for those I loved.

My reactions during that moment were no different than countless men and women serving our communities daily. Our reliance on remaining the strong foundation for others, portraying only stability and strength, causes us to enter and remain in a constant state of stability. This state is only bolstered by the fact that to put on the uniform and work the streets in the capacity of peace officer not only needs us to be strong, but it also requires it. Any outward signs of struggle or emotion would render us weak and hence display the opposite to a community which depends upon the strength we exhibit.

As described by Mark Malmin (2012) "the police subculture leads officers to feel that they need to act as though they can handle anything; it emphasizes individual strength and independence, which encourages personnel to maintain a façade of invincibility". Not unlike my response to my daughter, officers all around this great country and I would suffice to say our world, systematically learn to overcome emotion in an attempt not only of self-preservation but as a means to preserving societal stability and the avoidance of chaos.

Understanding fully the inner longing to serve with valor and strength, and to truly maintain the outward expression of what I truly felt inside, strength and the absence of any issues affecting me, I began thinking about it on a deeper scale. Fully understanding that there is a critical problem, with countless officers dying each day from suicide, the struggle is real. Feeling the stress and weight from the pure enormity of the job must take a toll, right? If so, why do most officers react consistently as I did? Why do we go about our day-to-day duties, like there was no problem? As I considered why many officers fail to seek help when struggling with the surfacing of long hidden trauma, I began a journey of taking the question to the source.

Although not conducting a formal study, each opportunity I came across fellow officers I would ask for their input. Describing to each of them that I was exploring the basic concepts of officer wellness and resiliency. I would simply ask my brothers and sisters why officers don't seek assistance when dealing with the stress related to their service. Listening to their responses predominately echoed my own answer to that question. In early 2021, the topic weighed heavily upon my mind. As I struggled to find the perfect method by which we could express our concern for our men and women in blue and get them to buy into reaching out for help, if needed, I began thinking about my journey. As I considered all the highs and lows, ups and downs of my career it dawned on me... I didn't need help and surely, they didn't either.

My deeply instilled belief, having been pounded into me from day one, was that I was strong. I was the stability my community needed, and the things I was seeing, and feeling were simply part of the job. Not unlike countless other men and women in the field we held the line and did it superbly. My citizens, friends, co-workers, family, and bosses needed me to simply do my job to the best of my ability and not worry about the residual garbage along the way. Perform admirably, treat everyone with respect, and preserve rights, that was what I was paid to do. The things I experienced, and the feelings I had inside, would simply have to be put to the back burner. All those things, those feelings, were simply part of the job and allowing them to affect me showed weakness. I truly felt that not giving those feelings or emotions a second thought worked out best.

The overwhelming majority of officers I speak to say the same thing. One of the major reasons officers fail to reach out is that, for the most part, our feelings and experiences are what we consider the norm. Our strength causes us to put away what we see and experience because it's all a part of the job. Why would someone reach out for help if they didn't think they needed it? Sure, we all know that officer, friend, or family member who could benefit from help. Many times, as we struggle to protect each other we may even talk to them about getting help. But in the end, we are good and any negative feelings we may experience are short lived and for the most part par for the course per se, because it's just what we do, overcome.

The deeply engrained tactic of remaining absent of emotion is truly a behavioral characteristic which is taught, reinforced, taught again, and repeated time after time throughout our training and our careers. In emphasizing the need to rid ourselves of emotion and not allow environmental stimulant to affect our responses, we in turn create within our communities a more stable, fair enforcement branch of the community. Think about those valiant officers standing strong on the front line of a protest. Being confronted with anger, disdain, and hate, many times, yet they remain stone faced and still regardless of whether citizens are screaming in their face or not. Does this image tell us anything about those serving in our communities? Is their response to external stimuli a reflection of stability or one of havoc? Stability, of course. Officers have from day one of their academy training been taught that their feelings, beliefs, and morals are secondary and not as important as that of the common good. This is an attribute which allows the officer to uniformly dispense law enforcement with fairness regardless of the situation.

Similarly, remaining somber and emotionless, the officer finds it within himself or herself to carry out their duties without consideration of any external factors such as race, gender, creed, or preference. I used to describe this aspect of police behavior to people desiring to enter the field of law enforcement with a simple interview question. Midway through each interview I would begin to get a good feeling of where the person stood on several social issues. Describing the importance of fair play, I would ask them a difficult, highly personal question. Sometimes I would ask about race related rallies and for others I would ask about pro-life rallies. I would describe that at times, as peace officers we are tasked with the duty to protect those whose core beliefs or motives are the opposite of ours. Asking young, wannabe cops, if they would be able to protect citizens whose views drastically differed from their own routinely came with a moderate amount of thought, unease, and ultimately an understanding that fairness was necessary on our fruitful society. Fielding a team of officers who relied upon their emotions and succumbed to feelings would lessen the effectiveness of the police force hence, engraining deep within each officer the importance of voiding ourselves of emotion is essential.

Emphasizing total control of emotion routinely continues throughout each day of an officer's career. The individual officer's ability to control their emotions and keep their responses in check sets the tone for not only their longevity within their career but likewise the quality of the same career. Over the years officers must learn that the job itself has very little to do with themselves but everything to do with those they serve. I routinely hammered this essential point home with junior officers through doing what I do best... telling them stories.

One such story I gladly relayed to them was about a spring day in the mountains of Colorado. I had just completed my lunch and while driving back to work I noticed a young lady walking alongside the roadway. As I drew close to the female, I immediately recognized her as a local girl who had an outstanding warrant for her arrest. Wishing I hadn't seen what I saw, I knew I had little choice but to engage the lady, even though I had the knowledge that she routinely could be found in a highly intoxicated and combative state. I pulled my marked patrol vehicle to the emergency shoulder of the road and approached the woman.

Upon approaching, she seemed very calm and collected. When I explained that she had a warrant commanding her arrest it all changed in an instant. In cop terms, the fight was on. This five-foot tall, ninety-pound lady gave this enormous monster of a man, gloating a sleek six-foot-seven frame everything he could handle right there alongside highway 119. Like a Hollywood B real movie with a flash of comedy, I was able to adequately control her and regain my dignity. Once I was able to get her restrained her combative nature physically subsided, but her verbal distain entered into an entirely new realm. Following securing her in my vehicle and notifying the dispatch center of our pending response to the jail, she missed no opportunity to voice her disgust for me and anyone else within ear shot.

As I drove this citizen with a vocabulary which caused the old sailor in me to blush, I simply remained calm and attempted to deescalate her with each passing word. It was then that the image of my mother and daughter caught her eye. As a young officer I found solace in a small wallet sized picture of the duo which I had placed in the driver's side visor of my vehicle. Unfortunately, the pictures calming effect were lost on the female and upon seeing it she simply asked, "is that your mom"? As I turned towards her, I simply replied "yes". Expecting my response, she then felt it necessary to describe to me that my mother was a street walker involved with prostitution. Although choosing a more modern, slang driven verbiage the woman's point cut deep. As I took a moment to breathe and center myself, I calmly turned, looked at the picture, turned back to the woman and replied, "dang it, I told her to stop doing that". Surprised that I didn't respond to her in anger the woman was taken back a bit. She looked at me, leaned back in her seat, and simply began laughing. The remainder of our drive was uneventful and communicative as I had broken through her barrier of anger through a bit of comedy.

As I have portrayed it hundreds of times, I had a choice in that moment. My choice was to respond in a manner void of anger. Sure, hearing someone say that my mom was a prostitute angered me. But what it all came down to was that she was going to jail, I was going home that night, and resorting to a negative response or action simply would have caused me and my career damage. The momentary satisfaction from my acting in a less than professional manner or saying what I really wanted to say would have been heavily outweighed by the negative ramifications for my actions if I had chosen to react in other ways. This, my friends, is what drives your law enforcement professionals many times.

Assisting our men and women wearing the uniform to reach an understanding that at times they may need help or may require a wakeup call relating to their emotional health is a difficult task. As stated, many are just like me, reluctant to allow the things I saw or experienced to affect who I was or would become. For a person to tell me that I needed help or was slipping into a dark place made no sense. I was secure in my abilities to maintain my composure and truly felt help was for the weaker guy, not me. What I found was the reluctance wasn't broken down until it was to late for me. I had become a perfect student of the game. Void of all emotion, ready at the drop of a pin to continue a life of service and sacrifice to my community. It truly was a shame that I had to be reminded from the lips of a nine-year-old little girl that my hesitation was having an effect on every other aspect of my being.

Chapter Summery and Key Takeaways

· Law Enforcement officers often hesitate to recognize the need for their own emotional wellness. This is due to multiple factors but primarily because of their deeply engrained belief that there is no need because they are fine.

· Law Enforcement Officers are taught early in their career that they must become void of emotion to ensure fairness and an equal distribution of the law.

· We as individuals have the ultimate choice of how we respond to verbal triggers. Our response can many times be indicative of our eventual longevity in the field and our ultimate career satisfaction.

Chapter Five

Common Issues for Law Enforcement

"We cannot solve our problems with the same thinking we used when we created them."

~Albert Einstein

As I began my law enforcement journey, I truly had no idea the impact it would have on me as an individual. Like many before me, I saw movies dedicated to the peace officers, watched television documentaries about crime and even did an ample amount of research into the field prior to entering in. The ideas of fame and heroism overshadowed any negative factors I learned about from friends and mentors. For me, I was becoming a member of a sorority of brothers and sisters destined to change the world for the better, protecting those less able from those intent on causing them harm. Upon dawning my uniform, I would instantly be transformed into the realm of savior, warrior, and hero. What I neglected to understand from all those conversations I had with experienced officers was the impact my chosen career would have on me emotionally and physically.

The life of any person holding the title of law enforcement official, or leader, follows a path that is directly similar in many ways to that of all others serving. Although differing in timing and in some cases severity, all men and women filling the shoes walk along the same proverbial path, hearing and seeing the same things albeit to differing severities. The fact that all officers encounter similar events and experiences throughout their career is an aspect which creates both a glimpse of potential for healing and a great barrier wall to progress, many times simultaneously.

The issues or experiences officers and leaders face encompass a great array of personal, environmental, and societal hazards many times possessing the potential of causing an accumulation of trauma. An accumulation many times not recognized and left untreated, or treated in makeshift ways to avoid truly coming to terms with the subject matter and experiences. The ultimate goal within the mind of police servants routinely is to increase sustainability within the police culture. This increase in sustainability is often accomplished through the use of humor within the police culture to offset the negative attributes they are experiencing.

For any outsider, the mere fact that officers would voice a quick joke or allow the conversation to turn dark, in the presence of a horrendous crime scene, death, or simply a bad scene where others had been hurt, causes alarm. Their shock and dissatisfaction relating to police responding in similar fashion is truly an example of how disengaged the public truly is in their lack of understanding of police culture. For the everyday law enforcement officer out there, the actions are merely their way, their brother's way, of coping with what they are experiencing, many times so they can sleep at night.

As described by Garcia, Nesbary, and Gu (2004) not only do the officers serving our communities deal with the trauma they see each day but the field in general adds to the stressors felt by officers. They describe "the top-ranked stressor for officers is a concern for fellow officers being injured or killed". The thought of a fellow officer being injured or killed is a heavy weight upon officers. I would gladly go out on a limb and assert that within the police community, the mass majority, if not all, officers are secure in their premise that they would without hesitation risk their own life to secure the life of a fellow brother or sister. Although an ever-present danger, the thought adds to the stress of those serving and their leaders.

I remember shortly after one of my own officers was severely injured in a shooting. I overheard a fellow leader, within the law enforcement community talking about how difficult the entire situation had been. As this competent leader spoke, he described that he couldn't do it. He revealed that he truly believed that if he was in that situation where one of his "guys" had been shot, he would have to "hang em' up" meaning he would cease being a police leader.

Although a major stressor, the threat of death or injury to oneself or a fellow officer, is unfortunately one of many negative events our men and women in blue face numerous days each day while serving the public. Mark Malmin, described in his article Changing Police Subculture (2012) "They will witness more sorrow, death, mayhem, and horror in six-months than many people will see in a lifetime." He went on to describe "nothing will prepare them for the first time they find a body hanging from a rope- nothing will erase the image of that event from their minds". The exciting, service-directed vision of policing that they began with is quickly replaced with the images flashing through their minds of the pain and sorrow felt by the wide array of victims they face with each new call for service.

The constant barrage of stressors and trauma leaves a wake of destruction behind as officers strive to continue their law enforcement journey. Many times, the effects of the constant stress are easily observable while at other times they remain hidden within the confines of the officer's mind. One of the more poignant examples of the effects of stress on officers as they progress with their career is what is routinely identified as the "Old Salt" or "Old Guy" syndrome. Within every police department and Sheriff's Office throughout our country a valuable group exists. Whether the department is framed by the beauty of the pacific northwest, the rugged dunes of New Mexico, the hills of the Ozarks or the hustle and bustle of the one of our major cities, the "Old Guy" finds a home. Routinely a police servant who has served for several years, the "Old Guy" is basically an unapproachable, angry man or woman, who simply wants to be left along to finish up his career in peace. There is nothing he or she hasn't seen, and they will gladly describe where the younger guy is falling short or making a mistake. Although remaining heavily committed to policing, the enormity of the job has routinely weighed upon the old guy and the damage is great, leaving them a shell of the person they once were, waking many nights with visions of death standing at along their bedside.

What is the natural progression from the excited recruit or "Newby" to the "Old Guy"? Each differs greatly. Some officers spend a lifetime within the career seldom feeling the effects upon their own person and avoiding the "old Guy" attitude while others rapidly fall victim to it. In both cases, the barrage of death, pain, rape, devastation, and simply general distain has visual effects on the officers. Effects which sometimes are rarely noticeable and at other times shine brightly like the beacon from a distant lighthouse. It is common within any law enforcement agency to see the effects of work-related stress.

Law enforcement officers who experience the day-to-day stress of the position and have an inability to or choose not to recognize or treat the damage routinely experience a wide array of behavioral changes which ultimately affect their lives not only at work but also outside of work. One of the most poignant effects continued, untreated stress has on the men and women serving is as I described earlier. The "Old Guy" syndrome or simply not caring anymore is prevalent. The untreated stress and day-to-day monotony of service creates a distain for everything and anyone around the officer. The officer descends into a chasm of despair where tiredness prevails, and the officer simply cannot pull themselves out of it. I found myself falling quickly into this same chasm late in my career, as I described in the original The Calling book. The events which surrounded me caused me to rapidly descend into unnavigated territory. Throughout my career, I routinely caught myself becoming depressed or overwhelmed. Using coping strategies, I was always able to pull myself up and get back to normal. This time it was different. For whatever reason I was unable to escape. I lived an existence where I didn't want to talk to anyone, I just wanted to shut my door and be left alone. Putting on the smile and welcoming demeanor had become difficult and many times impossible. I had become the one I said I never would, I had become the old guy.

The modern law enforcement officer often experiences a wide array of negative effects from the constant barrage of trauma. Although varying in enormity, the effects officers feel is truly real and unavoidable given the field. Being constantly confronted with external stimuli such as crime, suffering and angst, officers seldom can avoid the potential hazards and often succumb to the darkness of their career. This inability to overcome the external stimuli is many times the result of the traumatic event or crisis overwhelming one's normal coping strategies. Although common, a person's response to this overwhelming stimulus can surface moments later or even days or months in the future.

For law enforcement officers, how those emotions surface is far from stereotypical. For some, feelings of anxiety, guilt, panic and even uncertainty can prevail while with others, depression, nightmares, and making poor decisions is the result. For many viewing our officers at work, in their element of service, the possibility of recognizing the trauma surface is nearly impossible. Commonly, the result many officers feel from a buildup of stress related trauma exposes itself in many ways including an inability to sleep adequately. Not only can this danger be contributed to stress which results from trauma, but also in the mere position itself.

For law enforcement officers stable, consistent shifts work is purely a pipe dream, unachievable to most. The field routinely causes officers to engage in shift work anywhere from eight to twelve hours long. One week the officer may be assigned to a day shift and the next week to a night shift, so consistency is only a concept to be desired rather than obtained. Additionally, every law enforcement officer fully understands that the scheduled end of shift time is merely a recommendation because the officers are routinely tasked with varying their end time due to circumstances. The domestic violence call five minutes before the end of shift may be something some fields can put off for the next shift or avoid, but for law enforcement you can't. I cannot fathom the dates missed, money lost, scheduled shifted because I had to extend my go home time because of a crisis. Similarly, the field itself requires a quasi-seat of the pants response to planning all your time off.

When a crisis occurs, when tragedy strikes, the response of law enforcement cannot wait. Many times, depending on the severity, one's time off is affected by the need of their department to have them present and assisting. The ever present shifting of work times and the pure havoc of the position, one moment resting in pure boredom then without notice flying by the seat of your pants to highly stressful, life or death calls, takes a toll on the human body. All the aforementioned stressors can easily become the fuel which sparks potential health and emotional issues with officers.

In addition to sleep pattern disruptions officers face an expanding level of angst over their perceived lack of support from not only their communities but many times their direct supervision. As described in *Zhao, He, & Lovrich, 2002;* "Stressors in policing tends to view police organizational structures and various management practices as one of the primary sources of stress ". Organizational stressors combined with "perceived an increase in public scrutiny, adverse publicity, and perceived decline in police camaraderie" all contribute to officers experiencing a heightened level of stress according to the National Institute of Justice (2000).

The negative effects are not only felt by the officers themselves. Many times, police families succumb to work related stressors causing added difficulty to the officer him or herself. The general difficulty with planning and engagement due to shift work and overtime, an officer's inability or unwillingness to express emotion, fear for safety of their loved one, an inability to cope, and perceptions of their officer being paranoid or excessively vigilant can add to family related stress. As any person involved in family life knows, those stressors can easily enhance one's own personal stress and cause the individual to begin resenting loved ones and acting in a manner inconsistent to their norm.

It's not natural for a human being to experience the day-to-day trauma our law enforcement officials face routinely. This is precisely why officers, in hopes of coping, enter the belief system that they must void themselves of all emotion. For without emotion, we won't feel the pain associated with any given event and in turn be better equipped to carry on our duty as a safeguard. In many cases the officers become so well versed in the concept and fine tune their abilities that over time, the events simply become a part of the job and no longer hold any significant bearing upon the minds of those officers... so they believe.

Chapter Summary and Key Takeaways

· Unlike any other field, the role of law enforcement official carries with it a wide array of experiences, seldom felt by those outside the field. Although varying in severity, all officers are forced to engage in similar events which cause the officers to create coping mechanisms which are foundational to their sustainability in the field.

· Police officers will experience stressors stemming from their own personal safety, the safety of their co-workers, death, pain and suffering unlike any experienced by any other field.

· Work related stress can surface in a wide variety of ways including sleep disruption, marital/ family problems, cynicism, feelings of irritability or anger leaving the officer with a desire to simply avoid contact and many times react in a manner inconsistent with their normal response.

· A common coping strategy for officers is to resort to dark humor to deal with external stressors in their lives.

Chapter Six

Sliding into the Abyss

"This life. This night. Your story. Your pain. Your hope. It matters. All of it matters."

~Jamie Tworkowski

As I sat behind my desk, in the office I was so very proud of developing, I felt nothing but angst. Not unlike the flowing fields of winter wheat, moving with the breeze, my mind moved rapidly yet stationarily affixed to my ever-engulfing tiredness. A tiredness which overtook every aspect of my being. My thoughts seemingly remained tethered to an immovable object like a root system designed not only to support but likewise to hold in place. Unmovable and although supportive, my surface persona remained welcoming while crying out for solace within the deep confines of my mind.

When I was a sophomore in high school my dad accepted a position with a small country church on the eastern plains of Colorado. While excited, I experienced a great deal of concern over the move. I would be leaving the home, the schools, the friends I knew my entire life. I would go from a modern place where sleeveless shirts, Levis' and Addidas were prevalent and enter a realm where cowboy boots plaid shirts and the smell of livestock brewing in the heat prevailed. Repositioning myself within the local culture would be interesting to say the least but possible. Being a private person, delighting in privacy and often found playing by myself, I wasn't overly popular among my peer group, so the aspect of clique management wouldn't be an issue.

What I learned was once I gave the new area a chance, I would actually find myself thriving in this new location with these new friends. No longer was this lanky uncoordinated young man an outcast of sorts. That person had been replaced with someone who had opportunities to excel on many fronts. Residing in the Eastern plains allowed me to benefit from an agricultural culture, learning new and innovative ways to carry out routine tasks and overcome challenges which so often exist. No longer did I have to worry about simply blending in with the crowd, for my sheer size ensured I would always stand out.

My dad and I joked many times prior to his death about the belief that his good old son, all six foot seven of him was the reason he obtained the calling to pastor the church in Linden. I remember finding it strange when the church's pastoral search committee seemed to look me up and down, as I had a difficult time not catching their watchful eyes as we attended an interview lunch at a local restaurant. In the end, dad was hired, and the local school got a new basketball center, much taller than any other boys in the region.

Being the young man I was, I found little joy in academics but thrived off my newly found stardom with athletics. I would continue as I had throughout my life before the move and study little, rarely complete homework and hope only for a minimal passing grade to keep dad off my back. I remember this system of survival came to a screeching halt one afternoon when while preparing for that night's basketball game I was informed by my coach, Tom George, that I was ineligible due to academics. For me, it wasn't that big of a deal. Coach Georges' response was unsettling at the time and genius upon looking back.

Upon notifying me that I would not be playing ball that night, the coach explained that I would be seated on the bench with my team, in dress shirt, slacks and a tie. The thought of this was somewhat bothersome to me and could potentially cause some embarrassment in my mind. As I devised a plan to counter the embarrassment, I began to feel some relief. It was simple, if anyone asked, I would simply explain I twisted an ankle or pulled a muscle. That would appease the crowd's curiosity while maintaining my status of good student athlete. As any coach or parent does, I'm relatively certain Coach George sensed my lack of concern and added one more requirement. "Also", he grumbled, "if anyone asks you why you're not playing you are going to tell them the truth". Hearing this instantaneously caused a wave of worry and embarrassment to flow over by mind, body, and soul. Once recovering from the shock of hearing his words, I remained steadfast. I could simply limp a little and that would cause people not to ask. I would be ok after all.

Later that evening the true nature of my beloved Coach came to light. I had never had so many parents and community members walk up to me and inquire as to why I wasn't playing. It was truly a strange thing. With the coaches' words "tell em" The truth" repeating itself in my head, I had no other option but to be truthful, although embarrassed. It occurred to me later that my dear old coach had sensed my lackadaisical concern towards my grades, and he set out to make a point and shape my future. Prior to the game he approached several parents and asked them to ask me about why I wasn't playing, in effect accomplishing exactly what he set out to. I was never ineligible again.

What my coach imparted upon me was the importance of recognizing when the path we choose is counterproductive for us and rather than simply ignoring or making excuses about our failures, we must face them head on and deal with them in a positive manner. Sure, sometimes dealing with our issues can be embarrassing or disconcerting at times, the alternative of allowing the negatives to brew and eventually overflow can and will have lasting detrimental effects upon our future.

For me I knew all the right words to say and could easily recite positive coping strategies for my peers and personnel. It was like I was quick to save the men and women under me but slow to accept my own need. As I sat at my desk, the culmination of multiple years of unrelenting, constant, trauma and damage had finally come to a head. Not only was my work, relationships, and community involvement adversely affected, my faith was beginning to waver. For me personally, my family life never slowed. It seemed I retreated into their shield of protection and found it safe and inviting there. For many, they do not experience that same benefit.

I often wonder if one of the reasons I was unable to pull myself out of the depths of my struggle could be contributed to the loss of my father. Growing up, I was truly blessed to have a mountain of a man as my mentor. Not only was he a mountain in the physical sense, with his heavy, six-foot-four, broad shoulders, and firm chin ready and willing to protect those he loved. He came equipped with a rather large "preachers' belly" soft, yet supportive for the times I simply needed a hug. He also was a mountain in the sense of stature, stability, and wisdom. Rarely did I experience a time when I needed advice or leadership that he couldn't be found.

In 2017 we lost dad, and in losing him I lost my only truly safe outlet. Dad was the consummate family man. Old school by nature, his desire to provide for his family overshot just about everything in my early life. Although he would be gone for long periods of time as an over the road truck driver, we never went hungry. I remember he would routinely pawn his beloved rifles to simply provide milk when the times got tough. When dad felt the call of God to enter the ministry, he broadened his love to include the church and community as well. Settling in as the only son of the local preacher, doing my best to keep my elder sister in line, I always depended upon the fact that although extremely busy, dad could always be approached.

At the age of fifteen, our blessed little family would expand. While experiencing a moment of teenage laziness, I found myself sprawled out on the couch when mom and dad walked in. The words they said next not only excited me, but they also sent me into a zone of confusion because truthfully, the thought of mom and dad engaging in such behaviors was just plain wrong. They explained that I would soon have a younger sibling because mom was pregnant. The kicker to this notification was that following my birth, mom and dad, content with their son and daughter, had received a medical procedure ensuring she would no longer bear children.

My younger brother John would soon be born. Considered a blessing to mom and dad, because of the circumstances, I was content because although we had a baby at home my life changed minimally. Although dad loved each of his three children immensely, John held a special place in his heart. Maybe it was the fact that he was home more with John or maybe just dads core belief that God provided a miracle in their having John, either way, he was special. In March of 2014, John, his wife, and three of their children were killed in a motor vehicle accident, while returning home from a trip to Colorado. I recall the exact moment I had the unfortunate duty to notify mom and dad of their beloved sons' death. While mom wailed, dad remained somber and unable to speak or move. What transpired over the next two and a half years was truly an act of the ever-living God.

A short time following the burial of my brother we began seeing changes in dad. His ability to remember things, recognize acquaintances and recall scripture began deteriorating. As dads' doctors described he was suffering from dementia. They added that they had never seen a person slip from a totally normal state to a full on Dementia patient so quickly. Within a matter of months dad became totally dependent upon others and could only recognize me as a relative. As I sat wondering why such bad things happen to such good people, I experienced what was in my mind a moment of clarity.

Dad's experience was apparent to me, it was a genuine act of compassion from God. Many may disagree but my belief is mine and won't be changed. I believe dad experienced so much internal pain and suffering due to the loss of John that God found compassion upon him and wiped his mind away so he could stand up under the pain. Although dad held on for some time, I had the honor of repaying some of his lifelong commitment to me by looking into his eyes and allowing him to go home to his beloved son John. With a smile on his face, eyes firmly fixed upon mine he drifted off to heaven, a new man, made whole again by his Father in heaven.

As we shifted through dads' possessions, after his death, I remember my mother giving me his personal bible. For me, possessing the bible of generations of relatives has always been a quasi-hobby of mine. I find solace in the act of thumbing through the same pages my grandparents and great grandparents thumbed through, reading their notes and simply holding a item which they revered so adamantly. Holding dad's bible bore an extra special significance to me. As I opened the back zipper compartment, I was shocked to see a single picture inside.

As I removed the picture, my eyes watered a little as I gazed upon my senior picture, pristine, and unmarked after over thirty years. The picture in itself wasn't a huge thing for me, what bore more significance was its location in relation to the words my cousin spoke to me the year prior. While experiencing a down moment, I received a message from my long-lost cousin. After speaking for a bit, he relayed to me that he enjoyed his visit with my dad a year before he began experiencing dementia. In closing he described that dad was a good kind man and that he missed him greatly. He then said the words which cemented my understanding that my prior reasoning and beliefs were in error. He described "Rick, your dad told me how proud he was of you. He said, "you and you alone were his hero". It was at that moment that all my internal insecurities relating to my relationship with my father drifted away. Although undeserving, I made my dad proud.

The loss of this monumental outlet for me may have contributed to who I became during the waning days of my career in law enforcement. More so, I believe adamantly that a thirty-year career, putting all my burdens to the back burner, failing to address my trauma in a positive manner created a springboard of sorts. As with many men and women bearing the badge, unresolved trauma was left to simply build up. Building up to the point that it had no place to go but to overflow. For many this overflowing causes them to adjust their actions and inevitably causes them to act inappropriately, change behaviors, and fracture relationships. For some the overwhelming response to untreated trauma causes them to lose hope and engage in behavior counter- productive or in an unhealthy manner. To others, this loss of hope sends them reeling into a cavern of despair, finding no viable option but to harm themselves or end the suffering.

As described by Cristina Civilotti (2022) "Hopelessness is a particularly crucial condition and a risk for suicide". Going on, she describes that studies show twenty-six-point five percent of officers surveyed described hopelessness as being a major part of their lives and major contributor to burnout. Burnout is a syndrome according to Civilotti, that "results in chronic stress at work that has not been successfully addressed". Traditionally, burnout has been described as the three -dimensions of ex-exhaustion, cynicism, and depersonalization". For officers who consistently face work related trauma and fail to recognize the benefits of finding positive coping strategies, the result is similar to sinking deeper and deeper into an abyss destined upon total destruction. It is only through actively deciding to add a bit of preventative measures to our routine that true healing can be experienced.

Chapter Summary and Key Takeaways

· Recognizing when the effects of stress and trauma are beginning to affect us personally and socially is important. Likewise, engaging in positive measures to offset or counter the negative aspects of our careers and life is essential.

· External factors including loss or friends, or family members can many times set the tone for a loss of hope. This loss can heavily contribute to the emotions and traumas we have pent up deep inside to escape and spill over.

· Hopelessness and becoming burnt out are contributing factors when considering declining health. With 26.5% of officers surveyed describing feelings of hopelessness, proactive approaches must be implemented to offset the damage cause by work related trauma.

Chapter Seven

Time for Preventative Measures

"Each of us has a unique part to play in the healing of the world"
~Marianne Williamson

How our law enforcement officials and to be brutally honest, our first responders cope and or come to the realization that the trauma they experience on a day-to-day basis is beginning to overtake them and they are in need of assistance, is not unlike the way many people within the field and outside the field deal. Whether it is the cop, firefighter, military person, electrical worker, or preacher, we all experience stress on different levels. Sure, the enormity and amounts may very but its stress all the same. Stress which we often neglect and in the end are forced to confront the issue and decide to do a little preventative maintenance to ensure our sustainability.

For me, as described earlier, it was when I got to the point where I knew deep inside that I could no longer pull myself out of it. For years, I would recognize when the stress was building up and I would engage the normal coping mechanisms which had so faithfully pulled me up. I was faithful to ensure the accumulative stressors of the job weren't affecting my family. It wasn't until my normal strategies failed to render the result, I was accustomed to, and my beloved wife rocked my world with four simple words. One evening, while enjoying a quiet dinner, my wife described "you're never happy anymore". Those words caught me off guard. Although the one place I truly found happiness, my family, was always an aspect which demanded a simulated protective shield in my mind, they themselves felt my distance and the effects of my plight. This coupled with the fact that I had retreated into a realm of solace at work, preferring to simply remain in my office and not be bothered by anyone, demanded corrective action in my mind. What did that corrective action look like? I didn't know. But I knew it had to happen if I was to continue.

For others the revelation or needing help comes at a much greater cost. A longtime friend, co-worker, and brother in blue, Christian Martin, described:

There wasn't any one particular event that caused me to say to myself, hey, I need help. It was more of a slow burn to the end of a wick that I really had no idea existed. After many years in law enforcement, I no longer could deny the effects upon my mind, soul, and body of the traumas that I experienced. We are not wired to witness ten-year-olds commit suicide with their dad's belt from a bunk bed; we are not wired to process the weekly, if not nightly, fights that turn into a fight for our lives; nor are we able to successfully catalog horrific crash scenes where young people die in our hands.

The last several years of my career, I experienced vivid nightmares every night. I hated going to sleep. Even on my few days off I had during the week, sleep was elusive, and I never experienced a restful night's sleep. There were certain isles in the grocery store I could not walk down because of products which would trigger flashbacks that would cause me to see the face of a child I couldn't save, which was eating a certain item when he died. This was hard because I was the guy who used to think flashbacks were bogus.

Many other instances and triggers that I would deal with through the years from calls out of my control and I berated myself for having flashbacks and the anxiety they produced. I truly felt it was stupid that I was having such feelings, which only compounded the strain upon my mind. During the last few years as a police officer, I could not decompress and always operated in a hypervigilant state of mind.

I hated myself and was tired in my mind. The tiredness was unrelenting. As the years in law enforcement ticked by, I contemplated suicide every day, sometimes several times each day. I can't count how many times I rested my service weapon on my temple and did a press check, hoping it would go off. Shortly after I retired from law enforcement, my thirty-plus year marriage ended. I continued to have nightmares every night. Flash backs came frequently. Crowds were not doable as they caused great anxiety. Simply said, I hated people; I hated myself. I became extremely manipulative and harsh with those around me. After a second relationship fell apart, I came to the realization that there seemed to be some patterns I had developed. It was then that I realized, for the first time, perhaps some of what I was experiencing was because of Post Traumatic Stress. It was then that I decided to reach out for professional help.

Not unlike Christian, the lives, careers, and families of officers all around the globe are affected, many times adversely, by the years of trauma and a buildup of stress commonly found in the lives of those serving. Another officer described "I woke up one day and realized I was depressed and not feeling myself. Nothing interested me. I began having nightmares and didn't want to spend time with my family". For each officer the point that they come to the realization that they are experiencing a reaction to the daily trauma they confront is different. Like their individual reaction, the timing and what their experience entails is highly personal and rarely conforms to other experiences.

For some of those serving our communities, the recognition of feelings outside the norm is enough to vault them into help. For many others, their perceived stature, hero persona and self-derived stigmas hamper any attempts of recognition. It is many times the result of a total incapacitation of sorts when the officer finally comes to the point in their lives that reaching out for help is acceptable. Unfortunately, for many, the choice of help falls under a sinister action which forever ends their pain but in turn shifts that pain and struggle onto their loved ones. For those choosing to reach out for help and seek a little preventative maintenance of sorts, the future can once again brighten.

I first learned of the concept of preventative maintenance while working within the apartment industry shortly after returning home to Colorado after completing my service in the U.S. Navy. Fresh out of military service I remained somewhat unqualified to perform many of the high paying, highly desirable jobs I had envisioned. Raising a young family, the opportunity to begin working at the state's third largest apartment complex was a win-win for my family and I. Not only would I learn a great trade, but my monthly rent was also included so we had a roof over our heads and food in our bellies. Starting as a groundskeeper, I quickly moved up the food chain per se and after merely one year, sat in the maintenance supervisor's seat.

Grasping little about the maintenance field, I relied upon my leadership skills to make my way as the leader of a small work center ensuring that nine-hundred-fifty-seven apartments were maintained and operational. As the time passed on, I learned to rely on the wisdom of those who had spent a lifetime in the field. I remember one employee who was blessed to have a firm grasp of heating and ventilation. As he performed his daily tasks, he would consistently remind me about the importance of scheduling preventative maintenance. He described the mere act of routinely changing filters, cleaning machinery, and simply taking the time to make the machineries job easier would in fact lesson our need for emergency maintenance in the long run.

Not unlike the boiler driven heating system or the forced air unit, our bodies require a certain measure of preventative maintenance, to perform as intended. Coming to the point of realizing that maybe we overdid it or neglected the routine maintenance on our mind and body is more difficult but similarly crucial. I have always been a guy who simply becomes busy with life. Whether it is changing my oil, replacing air conditioner filters, or making sure the house has a new coat of paint, I often think about completing the tasks but quickly push it to the back burner to ensure I can complete the wide array of more important tasks.

Similarly, my life as a law enforcement officer and supervisor mirrored my personal responsibilities. I recognized many of the stressors I faced. Many times, I made a mental note that they needed addressed. But like changing the oil in my wife's car, it could wait because truly what harm could result from my waiting another week or two? The problem remains. It's not the simple act of failing to change the intake filter on the air conditioner unit. It's the buildup of debris on the coils, and the lack of air flow because of the clogged filter. Similarly, it's not simply the pushing to the back burner our trauma but rather the buildup of the trauma which many times can result in a breakdown in our ability to cope effectively.

True strength rests upon realizing and acting upon the need for change. I remember struggling to maintain a welcoming spirit while performing my duties my last couple years. Putting on the strong face, being the supporting shoulder, I would routinely lay aside my own personal feeling to ensure I was not only ready but likewise willing to extend an arm of support for my team when they were struggling. I have always been quick to give advice while simultaneously slow to apply the same advice I dished out.

Two instances of officers getting to the point of realization that something needed to change stood out to me and if I am being perfectly honest, haunt me to this day. The first was a young officer of mine who had recently gone through a horrid break up from a major relationship. I remember thinking to myself that break ups happen, and they really needed to suck it up even though the pain was real, because she would survive in time, just like I and countless others have. Because of the officer's youth, I approached the situation a little differently.

Feeling concerned because the officer hadn't been heard from in a few days, I responded with a fellow supervisor to their home where we contacted my officer. We found the officer, one of our sisters or brothers, seated on the couch, in a darkened house, struggling with their thoughts alone. As we spoke, it was apparent that my officer was in a bad spot.

Regardless of my experiences, or the experiences of others, what they were feeling was not only real but unique to them, and them alone. Understanding the gravity of the situation, I simply took the time to console.

Later, after explaining that I needed them to come hang out with their police family for a while, the officer agreed and my concerns were somewhat minimized at that point because they would be with their co-workers and not alone. I later found out from the officer that the dark place they were in at that time was causing them to see no way out. Being alone with their thoughts did nothing more than cause the pain from a lifetime of abuse to surface alongside their present feeling of despair, leading them to consider ending their life. Through the help of counselors and true friendship the officer prevailed and was able to recognize the need to maintain their wellness in spite of any inerrant stigma affixed.

The second memorable account occurred one day as a friend and brother in the mission approached me with an embarrassed look on his face. This man had walked alongside me through many times of trials and turbulence. Similar to me, he routinely put on the leaders' face and simply carried on. On this particular day, he stood before me, face down, shoulders folded, describing that he needed help. As we spoke, my friend described that he was having problems sleeping and experiencing nightmares. As I encouraged him and provided him with a moderate amount of praise for stepping forward, my mind began transitioning to a realm of embarrassment myself.

My embarrassment and borderline anger didn't stem from the statement of need from my friend or even an inner feeling of letting him down, because I had not. My feelings of anger were simply a reflection of my concern over his statement coupled with the statement from another deputy who had been injured in a shooting incident who had come to me saying "I'm sorry". When I heard this, I inquired as to why he was sorry and the words he said were simply words we should never hear in this modern world.

Somberly, my deputy described that he was sorry because he thought he had post-traumatic stress disorder stemming from the incident he was involved in. He was confused because he was strong, resilient, and trained. The problem was his demons were rapidly overtaking him.

One officer described it this way:

I hated myself and was tired deep in my mind, all the time. As the years in law enforcement ticked by, I contemplated suicide every day, sometimes several times a day. I cannot count the number of times I put my service weapon to my temple and did a press check, hoping it would go off.

Shortly after I retired, my thirty plus year marriage ended. I continued to have nightmares every night. Flashbacks came frequently. Crowds were not doable. I hated people; I hated myself. I was extremely harsh in criticizing others and became emotionally manipulative. After some internal work to fix some things, I got into a long-term relationship which eventually came crashing down. At that point I realized there were patterns I had developed, and for the first time I realized that perhaps some of what I was experiencing was because of PTSD. That's when I reached out for professional help.

As law enforcement administrators we must pave the way for every officer, first responder, and fire fighter to seek help without experiencing a feeling of angst or embarrassment. The men and women serving under me had nothing to be sorry about. And their reaching the point in their lives that they feel the need to seek help should be celebrated rather than cause them to hesitate or bare negative feelings about their own wellness. We must invite preventative maintenance within our pack and in ourselves.

Chapter Summary and Key Takeaways

· Law Enforcement officers reaching the point of realization that they may need help is as unique as the officers themselves. Some officers reach those points quickly, some only after years of trauma.

· Reaching that point of realization or need for some comes only after a total breakdown in their ability to cope and for some after a singular incident.

· The symptoms of overwhelming trauma differ from officer to officer.

· Preventative maintenance is designed towards addressing potential stressors and making the necessary repairs in order to experience long term success and workability.

· Law Enforcement administrators must make reaching out for help the norm rather than an area of embarrassment or vulnerability for their peers and subordinates.

Chapter Eight

Countering the Damage

"In the end, we will remember not the words of our enemies, but the silence of our friends."

~ Martin Luther King Jr.

O nce our law enforcement officers, fire fighters, or other first responders get to the point of realizing that there exists a need they then must begin doing everything in their power to counter the damage. Many times, the realization for officers' stems from eclipsing that rock bottom, low point in their lives where the loss of relationships, positions, rank, or status is the result of failure to act upon the trauma. Many others fully understand that something is wrong but are unable to pinpoint the reasoning for why they are feeling the way they are and hence remain oblivious to the cause and eventual affect. In some instances, it is not the officer himself or herself who opens the proverbial door but the officers' friends, family, or co-workers. Regardless, a proactive series of countermeasures must be undertaken to ensure resiliency and longevity for the affected officer.

One of the most effective and proven successful manners by which to counter the damage from a lifetime of un-addressed trauma within the law enforcement community is simply affecting the culture through which each officer interacts with his or her public, brothers, and supervisors. As we have discussed not only in the original *The Calling: Seated at the Table with the Broken* book; but likewise in the earlier chapter of this offering, creating a culture of inclusion and acceptance within the modern police culture is essential. Given the barrage of factors pushing against a officer obtaining assistance including stigma, feelings of grandeur, super hero complex, and concern over the possible departmental and personal ramifications stemming from their seeking help, their reluctance is huge.

For many, the thought of seeking help regardless of the manner by which it is administered is eternally welcome and bears with it minimal negative ramifications. This factor can be seen through the barrage of feel-good commercials and movie scenes which flood our modern television. Scenes where full-grown men and women openly talk about their problems, lend a shoulder to cry on, and smile at the possibility of helping another through their latest stressful encounter at the local coffee shop. This assertion couldn't be the furthest from reality as I think about my brothers and sisters in blue.

Our law enforcement officers, as described, seldom feel the need to seek help, often not reaching that point of realization until they are so far gone, the damage is viewable by others and all options of reversal spent. Once they reach that point, honestly the last thing they want to do or feel the need to do is reach out to anyone let alone a behavioral health professional who is there to help rewire their errant thoughts. Not only does the untreated trauma, the officers have pushed aside for years, cause high levels of stress and other potentially deadly disorders, the damage caused by the thoughts of being at the point in their lives where seeking help is not only needed but required can cause debilitating stress and add to the officers feeling of confusion and concern.

I sat listening to a speaker several years ago who laid it out in a manner which was simple yet totally off point in my opinion. This speaker described that we had to do everything in our power to constantly remind officers about how much we cared for them and wanted them to get help. They assured everyone in the room that making officers accountable for their wellness would in turn create a stronger force of officers. They went on to describe that officers understand that there are no negatives associated with seeking help and hence our reaching out merely erects a bridge of sorts. As I listened, I will admit, I found it very difficult to keep my mouth shut and not openly disagree. For a man, deeply engrained in the police culture I fully understood the effects of what this person was asking. The effect of an in-your-face confrontation surrounding officer wellness and stigma.

Although I'm sure the speaker's intent was noble, the strategy had several fatal flaws. First, confronting an officer in an openly accusatory manner will get you absolutely nowhere. Lest we forget, many of these officers feel no need for assistance because to the crux of the issue, in their mind, they aren't struggling, they are doing what they are duty bound to do and dealing with the horrors they see is simply a part of it. Secondly, we cannot forget that officers have a deeply engrained belief that seeking help reveals weakness and weakness loses respect and confidence. Finally, the concern over ramifications for seeking help is real and reasonable.

I remember the first time I described to a behavioral health professional the fact that officers hesitate to speak to professionals within the mental health community because of a fear of "losing their gun". The look of utter shock and disbelief on the friends' face was shocking. As we spoke, I remember describing to my behavioral health friend that our approach on breaking down the stigma in all reality needed to go far beyond the officer him or herself. Truthfully, the minds of police administrators and our high-level politicians had to first be convinced of the need to rid ourselves of stigma.

As my friend continued to look bewildered, he simply asked me why I thought that and how or why would an officer be concerned about losing their weapon. As I began explaining that current federal law prohibits anyone who has been subject to certain mental health diagnosis to possess firearms, my friends face turned to confusion. "Really?" he said. As I continued, I described that to truly understand our officers we must first understand their fears. I asked my friend to think for one moment; think about having a career where possessing a weapon is not only required but many times pertinent to your survival. I elaborated, now think about working that job for years and for the most part knowing nothing else but the job because you have spent years putting your blood sweat and tears into that job. The job has seen you through ups and downs, seen relationships change and families grow. Now you ask them to risk all of that to step forward and "seek help", when they know deep down, they are messed up because of the same job they love.

As my friend stood in silence, it was apparent I had succeeded in taking him to a greater level of confusion. He responded simply, "wow, will they really take their gun?" The conversation unfortunately wasn't my first regarding this topic area. Since becoming heavily involved in the behavioral health community it was seemingly a major educational point. I was routinely met with disbelief and skepticism each time I relayed this fear to others. In some cases, people outright refuted my assertion. In the event that a behavioral health professional refused to understand the fear on the officers' part, I would simply ask them to do a little research. Helping them with their research, I invited them to check into the true-life story of one of our fellow law enforcement brothers, Chris Prochut, a former officer with the Bolingbrook Police Department in Illinois.

What these professionals will encounter, upon researching the fears of officers, is the reality of the concern whether we want to believe it or not. For Chris, his struggle with the stressors of the profession peaked when he was the face of the Bolingbrook Police Department during the Drew Peterson investigation. With the stressors seemingly growing daily, Chris describes that he got to a point where he was no longer able to contain his thoughts of suicide, even setting the date which he would take his own life. Through the intervention efforts of his wife and fellow police administrators his attempt was stopped, and Chris received behavioral health treatment. Because of that treatment and Chris's condition the state of Illinois revoked his ability to own or possess any firearm, for all practical purposes, rendering his career and the life he knew and loved worthless.

Luckily, the breaking down of stigmas associated with behavioral health and law enforcement has become a major point of emphasis throughout our society and the opinions and laws are seemingly changing to mirror the concern over breaking the stigma associated with seeking assistance.

As we consider truly affecting change, we must first grasp an understanding that there is no known cookie cutter, one size fits all approach to improving the wellness and overall resiliency of our law enforcement personnel. For some, the traditional therapeutic response proves itself crucial to healing and to others, the thought of sharing their story with a stranger is the furthest from their mind and pointless. Many officers find relief through peer groups and /or one-on- one conversations with trained individuals who walk the same walk, day in and day out, understanding the plight of the American officer. While others find relief in less conventional means of coping such as writing, exercise, and hobbies.

Many officers rely heavily on what I like to call the faith factor; their personal faith when dealing with the stressors of their chosen career. Each officer's choice to confront their proverbial demons is not only highly personal, but they are also systematically beneficial given the officer's choice to truly become engaged in their wellness. Regardless of the manner by which the officer chooses to bring the trauma to an end, the mere act of acting sets the tone for not only learning but overall success.

One officer I have had the pleasure of working alongside over the years described:

My reasoning for wanting to get into law enforcement is what almost broke me, almost ended my career, and ultimately got me back to the right frame of mind to stay in the career. Being the victim of childhood sexual abuse, I wanted to go into law enforcement as a career to stop what happened to me from happening to others. Once I was firmly ingrained in the field, I entered into a serious relationship which fell apart around the same time I was working on several child sexual abuse cases. I began having reoccurring nightmares about the abuse

I had been subjected to. The nightmares were so vivid and real. I made a huge mistake not finding someone to talk to about my problems. My refusal to get helped resulted in my having thoughts about killing myself. I struggled daily to simply continue on.

Realizing that my thoughts and stress was affecting my job I spoke to my supervisor who managed it the correct way. Rather than firing me as I envisioned, he provided me with time off for my mental health treatment and suggested several mental health professionals which I could begin seeing for help. Not finding a mental health professional I trusted, I simply gave up. I know this isn't the right answer, but it was my reality. I know I would have benefited from their help, but I just never felt comfortable.

It wasn't until I attended a Crisis Intervention Team Training a few years later, that I realized the importance of personally being accountable for our mental health. The training helped me gain a much wider perspective of mental health and how helping others deal with their own mental health in turn helped me deal with my own.

Countering the damage of trauma must be every citizen's emphasis and bear great significance to each of us. Regardless of whether it's trauma from the daily regimen of our careers or childhood trauma, tucked away, ensuring that effective coping mechanisms are in place is essential. As described, each officer is different and the manner by which those officers can effectively obtain treatment will differ. The key is simply that we pave the path to recovery utilizing every possible solution known to man to counter the damage.

Chapter Summary and Key Takeaways

·   The counter measures we deploy to effectively impede damage associated with trauma must be erected to enhance officer resilience. The most effective manner of countering the damage is to affect the culture by which officers reside within.

·   There is no one size fits all solution to officer wellness and resiliency. Each individual can find solutions which are highly personal and effective to them personally.

·   Numerous factors work against officers seeking help for their mental health. Stigma, validation, and fears must be addressed to reach our desired outcome of ensuring officers have the tools necessary to take control of their wellness.

Chapter Nine

Signs that it's Time

"The bad news is time flies. The good news is you're the

pi-

lot."

~ Michael Altshuler

For many, reaching the point of understanding that the things we are feeling or the experiences we are hearing in our mind and body can be frightening. For others, the thoughts and actions are merely hidden away from the rest of the world, behind the protective shield we have erected for self-preservation. Understanding why things are happening and why we are feeling the way we are is the first step to healing. I wanted to take a brief moment to get down to the nitty-gritty about mental health and describe some of the characteristics of stress and post traumatic symptoms. We explore this aspect of behavioral health with the full intent to broaden our understanding, so we are better prepared to recognize when and if the trauma we have been placing on the back burner is beginning to re-surface within our lives.

For me, although fully understanding the signs of depression, stress, and anxiety in others, I had a difficult time grasping their relation to me personally. As I described earlier, I was strong and could handle stress, so my duty was to protect my pack. It wasn't until the signs began overwhelming me that I came to the full understanding of behavioral health in relation to officer wellness. Many times, officers find it difficult to step outside the proverbial box, a concept they trained heavily upon, but rarely apply. The failure in my opinion is simply another force field or shield erected to maintain continuity with their strongly held belief that they are truly society's protector and as described by Stephanie M. Conn (2018) "the last true crime fighters."

What each of us must remember, as we commit to breaking down the walls of resistance and stigma within the police culture, is that we are dealing with a warrior class of individuals. Regardless of our feelings of the accuracy or error of that mentality it is alive and well within the police culture. Accordingly, the words of Neily, 2016, describe the plight superbly as they state, "from the initial event, where you may be fighting for your very survival, you must learn to transition to the ongoing fight for your well-being down the road". Not unlike my early days in law enforcement when I was driven to study case law in hopes of broadening my understanding of the law and enhancing the skills I could use on the job as I became determined to survive each day, our ability to understand the signs that our bodies and mind are feeling the wear and tear of time is essential.

Having an accurate understanding of the human body's typical reaction to stressors coupled with understanding and support of friends and family can "make a big difference to people affected by traumatic events" (ICISF, 2020). The manner by which a person reaches that understanding is not only essential but likewise different in many cases. There is seemingly no easy, non-textbook format available today which spells out the symptoms we may face. Until now. Over the next few pages of this offering, I will attempt to bring the issue to our readers in a down-to-earth and simple format in hopes that we can all benefit from it. Understand that this attempt towards understanding stems from a non-clinical, lifelong cop, so although accurate, my friends in the behavioral health community will have to bear with lack of "medical terms" and descriptions.

As we know, Law enforcement officers as well as other first responders routinely experience a wide array of external stimulus, daily, which can impact the quality of life they experience. Many times, the result of the trauma they experience is one or multiple possible behavioral health disorders. Many officers, young and old, described the effect of work-related stress and trauma on their person as debilitating. Commonly, disorders associated with post traumatic stress, depression, anxiety, and the spiritual impact of the job effects officers.

Post-Traumatic Stress

For someone to meet the criteria for post-traumatic stress a person has to be exposed to actual or threatened death; serious injury; sexual violence either directly or witnessed; and or experienced repeated exposure to aversive details of a traumatic event as a first responder (Conn, 2018). Commonly, the symptoms which follow these events or experiences include distressing memories, dreams, flashbacks, re-experiencing / reactions when exposed to environmental cues or reminders. A person's response to the feelings, thoughts, and actions associated with traumatic events can differ greatly.

For many officers who have experienced post-traumatic stress, the reactions and longevity can many times be indicative of an actual diagnosis of having a post-traumatic stress disorder. As one officer explained "I just wanted to be by myself because the memories wouldn't leave me alone". I recall early in my career speaking to one of those stereotypical "old timers". An officer with the Denver Police Department who mentored me as I entered into law enforcement. One statement he told me ended up being the one thing I could never lay aside, and routinely thought about. Pat described that early in his career he was involved in a shooting where a young boy was killed. Although the officer was fully justified, he described to me that every night he wakes up seeing the boy standing at the foot of his bed. Why did this simple story cause me so much thought? I don't know but have zero doubt that the incident itself seared itself in the mind of my friend for over twenty years.

Although the rates of post-traumatic stress amongst law enforcement typically aligns with the general public, the fact that our law enforcement officers who suffer from post-traumatic stress and then must continue to experience stimuli on a daily basis, makes the situation much worse. Simply put, our officers cannot escape.

Anxiety

It has been difficult for medical professionals, scholars, and practitioners to pinpoint the actual rates of anxiety within the police culture. One of the most common mental health conditions, anxiety, would automatically be considered a potential issue for law enforcement given the fact that although many fail to recognize the fact, our police are human as well. The mere fact that law enforcement engages in specific situations which breed anxiety, their exposure and interactions can open the door to a broader diagnosis.

In her book titled, Increasing Resilience in Police and Emergency Personnel (Conn, 2018) describes that "in a nutshell anxiety is fear relating to certainty (lack of), control, and comfort". The fact that our law enforcement officers face uncertainty on every level each day adds to the impact of anxiety on our lives. Let's think about that for a moment. Within the realm of policing, rarely does an officer feel certain of outcomes or even the one place they should be able to find solace, their department. Political upheaval and change can leave officers uncertain of their longevity at their desired place of employment. Additionally, the mere act of enforcing the law in certain areas or with certain individuals can be stressful for officers. I recall a young officer feeling frustrated because of his act of issuing a citation to a deserving citizen. Within moments that citizen contacted his cousin who happened to be on the board of alderman, the cousin called the mayor who called the chief, all pressuring the officer to rescind his deserving action.

Likewise, the lack of control officers feel is rarely pertaining to their job itself. Their fear or anxiety as they pertain to outcomes are normally less because of the work they are performing or the danger of street work but often times more accentuated by the shifts they are working, overtime, court appearances, and their perceived lack of influence over departmental policies. Comfort, the final tier of fear where anxiety is concerned, is somewhat a no brainer. To anyone who understands law enforcement, the comfort level in policing is truly non-existent. Regardless of whether it is being called in to work during your off time, asked to work late, working under adverse conditions, the job is far from comfortable. Officers, daily, face uncomfortable situations in environments which would cause the strongest to shriek in bewilderment. The long hours, uncomfortable gear, demeaning attitudes and fervent adherence to the rules cause their comfort level to plummet many times.

Depression

Some areas of research have depicted that law enforcement officers have a higher level of depression due to the environmental factors surrounding their duty (Violanti & Drylie, 2008). In many studies, we learn that more officers suffer from depression than post-traumatic stress. Depression itself is a confusing and somewhat stigmatizing disorder because many people truly question the legitimacy of the disorder. I have caught myself dealing with friends and family who suffer from depression, saying, to myself, get over it, you have a good family, job, and children who love you. What I had to learn was that for these loved ones, they couldn't "just get over it". For many people, officers included the thought of being depressed brings forth uneasy feelings of inadequacy. Some people feel that if a person is depressed, they are weak and can't handle the basic things in life. This assertion couldn't be furthest from the truth in my mind.

One of the most vivid examples of the impact of depression was in my own mother's life. Shortly after the death of my brother, then my father, my mom fell hard into a state of depression. Although she would most likely never admit it because she had lived a lifetime of strength and mentoring, she simply had a difficult time dealing with all the losses she was experiencing. The loss of our beloved family coupled with the ever-increasing number of she and dads' good friends who were passing away caused mom to desire nothing more than to lay down and sleep. Her sleep provided much needed comfort and relief from her thoughts and pain.

For some officers, mom's story is truly the description of their own lives. For officers, the barrage of negativity, death, pain, and suffering we see on a day-to-day basis leads them into a mode of depression. Let me ask a question of my fellow officers reading this today... how negative is your outlook? And how has your view of our world been impacted by your job? I would suffice to say that each officer answering described that their view is primarily negative and has been negatively impacted by our work in law enforcement. It's difficult to avoid. No other career places men and women in the forefront of negativity as law enforcement does. Although easily the foundation for depression one must understand that being depressed doesn't not necessarily mean the officer is at the point of being diagnosed with a full-blown depressive disorder.

Spiritual Impact

An officer's spirituality or faith many times lays the foundation for their day to interactions with others. As we discuss the concept of spirituality or faith, in this chapter and later in chapter fourteen, we first need to understand that where law enforcement resilience and overall wellness is concerned, I am not speaking of any particular religion, faction, belief system, or world view, but rather the concept of faith in something. Whether your faith is in God, Muhammad, Buddha, The Earth, or your family, an officers ability to maintain sight of their given faith can many times be the bridge between successful resilience and struggle. Faith is a extremely personal concept to each man and woman serving their community and must be not only valued but considered when searching for solutions.

As described by Websters Dictionary, faith is the "complete trust or confidence in someone or something". For the officer on the street, many times, the only relief they experience as they confront the evils of this world is their firmly held beliefs. Unfortunately, the job itself impacts one's faith many times. As described in one study on cumulative stress, "fifty-three percent of officers reported that their faith or religious beliefs had changed due to the job" (Marshal, 2003). How or why does this happen? Few know or understand. Maybe it's because most young men and women enter the field with high hopes of making an impact. What they often find is a non-supportive public, suffering, violence and corruption on all levels.

A field once considered noble and honorable has at times been replaced with feelings of anger and embarrassment with each incident of abuse of authority and death, at the hands of a fellow brother or sister acting not out of duty but rather out of self, viewable on the nightly news. The impact of police life can adversely affect officers' sense of connectedness which is a major factor with spirituality and faith. The day-to-day rigors of the field cause officers to want to disconnect with the communities they serve and fall back into a shell of connecting only with the pack.

One interesting fact surrounding spirituality and faith as it relates to law enforcement service is the understanding that in many cases, the faith of officers is emboldened by their experiences. As officers seek to find meaning in what they are experiencing or dealing with many times that meaning is found in their faith. The same faith becomes the foundation for how the officer deals with his or her stressors and their interaction with others.

When confronting trauma, throughout the day, many officers begin a process of thinking in ways which can not only be counterproductive but also lead to a worsening of the overall situation. Thinking purely "Black or White", the act of identifying people and events as only good or bad or right or wrong lends itself to neglecting the fact that in many instances the gray area is far more accurate and palatable. Likewise, jumping to conclusions, emotional reasoning, labeling, personalization, should have or could haves, and discounting the positives, although common, as we attempt to cope, can cause us to camouflage the true issues at hand and bypass effective resolution.

As many of us can relate, it is easy for an officer to fall victim to the afore-listed styles of communication. Officers tend to fight back the urge to see everything in the realm of black and white. It becomes easier to succumb to the process with each passing call. The difficulty which arises is the need to not only establish a common, positive, manner of viewing our world but likewise to avoid the mannerisms and habits of faulty thinking.

As officers carry out their duty to the public it is important to understand that although in many cases, avoiding, not succumbing to post traumatic stress, depression, anxiety or negatively affecting one's spirituality is impossible given the horrors we routinely see, recognition and countering the effects of stress is crucial. Recognizing when we may be experiencing one of these disorders can be a daunting task so I wanted to take a moment and list several possible indicators that we may be in trouble. My hope is that if we recognize that we are experiencing one or more of the symptoms that we seek to research how we can effectively counter the negative effects of stress.

Common Symptoms Immediately Following a Traumatic/ Crisis Event(s)

Physical

- Sleep Difficulties- Falling asleep or staying asleep
- Headaches
- Body Aches
- Nervous Energy – Need to be moving
- Heightened Startle Response
- Loss of Appetite
- Elevated Blood Pressure
- Nausea
- Dizziness
- Diarrhea
- Indigestion
- Chills

Cognitive

- Racing thoughts
- Confusion
- Intrusive Thoughts and Images
- Nightmares
- Forgetfulness
- Making careless Errors at Work
- Difficulty Making Decisions
- Blaming
- Hyper-vigilance
- Difficulty Calculating
- Time Distortions
- Auditory Distortions

Relational

- Withdrawal from family, coworkers, colleagues
- Withdrawal from organizations or affiliations
- Isolation
- Unemployment
- Discontinue educational pursuits.
- Lack of community and political involvement

Emotional

- Angry

- Sad
- Afraid
- Irritable
- Lost
- Numbness
- Shock/ Disbelief
- Depression
- Panic
- Lack of interest in normal activities
- Crying
- Guilt
- Uncertainty
- Irritability
- Anger
- Euphoria
- Obsessiveness

Behavioral

- Withdrawal from others
- Escape behaviors- Drinking, Shopping, internet surfing
- Increased risk taking
- Change in Speech
- Emotional Outburst
- Inability to rest.
- Pacing
- Change in sexual function/ drive
- Ritualistic Behavior
- Excessive spending

Spiritual

- Questioning beliefs
- Anger at God
- Loss of meaning
- Withdrawal from faith and religion
- Redefining moral values
- Promising, bargaining, or challenging God

Following a crisis or traumatic event it is common for people to experience strong reactions. Many times, those reactions and the person's response can be overwhelming to the person's ability to cope. The thought that a person will experience these reactions immediately is errant. Many times, our reactions can come minutes, hours, weeks, or even months in the future. Similarly, the person's reaction or symptoms can last days, weeks and in some cases even longer in duration. While understanding that different people react differently to trauma, the important thing is that we understand that stress effects people differently and the fact that they are experiencing a response to their stress does not symbolize a lack of strength or an inability on the persons part to serve their community and do their job. Simply said, it means they are human and must effectively utilize coping strategies.

There are many strategies to counter the damage of stress available today. Some of the most effective strategies can be completed utilizing the officer's most effective coping strategy, his or her family and friends. A broad support network, although simplistic by nature, has proven to make a huge difference to people affected by traumatic stress. Additionally, many proactive tools are believed to help. Below are several tools and strategies people who have become effected by traumatic stress can utilize to enhance their ability to cope:

- Spend the first 24-48 hours physically exercising and relaxing.
- Keep busy by structuring your time.
- Don't label yourself as flawed or "crazy". What you are feeling is normal.
- Talk to people. Talking is one of the most effective healing strategies.
- Reach out, people care.
- Maintain a normal schedule.
- Spend time with others.
- Help others by sharing your feelings.
- Avoid numbing your pain with alcohol or drugs.
- Give yourself permission to feel like crud.
- Keep a journal and write.
- Do things that feel good to you.
- Avoid making big life changes.
- Take back control of your life by making decisions and bringing back control in your life.

·   Don't try to fight re-occurring dreams, they are common and should decrease over time.

·   Eat a well-balanced diet.

I remember listening one day as one of the old guys, sitting just outside my door explained to one of our newly recruited kids (recruit officer) that there were several things he had to look forward to over the next several years. The recruit, wide eyed and excited about graduating the academy and starting work, listened intently as this mountain of a man began. You will lose all your hair son, look around at how many old guys have no hair. Likewise, you will lose that athletic build because fast food and the doughnut house is your easiest option. He then looked at the kid and said and worse than all of that "this job will steal your soul son" so be prepared. The kid, no longer in a mode of excitement, shook his head and simply replied "frickin old guys" and walked away with a smile.

There is a good amount of truth to the old guy's statements. Many in the field loose our hair and gain a waistline many of us aren't proud of. Losing our soul as the officer described was an analogy about how the field itself often strips us of all our previous beliefs, thoughts, and thoughts of mankind. Is the losing of our soul a given? No, but it is a difficult result which is difficult to overcome.   Any officer, if they are willing to honestly answer would describe a decline in their faith in humanity and community after several years of policing. Luckily, the opportunity to counter those thoughts and feelings associated with the day-to-day trauma we experience has become forefront in our desire to lift our brothers and sisters out of the valley.

Chapter Summary and Key Takeaways

·   Understanding the symptoms of traumatic stress is crucial to our survival.

·   Many members of the law enforcement community experience post -traumatic stress, depression, anxiety and spiritual questions because of the trauma which impacts their lives.

·   The symptoms of traumatic stress differ in duration and often vary. Experiencing symptoms is common and does not mean the individual experiencing them is flawed or broken in any way.

·   There are several common strategies which have proven effective in countering traumatic stress.

Chapter Ten

Conventional Methods- Therapy

"There is a solution to every problem. I just have to find the right solution to fix the problem."

~Brock Lesnar

Hearing the words "I think I need help" coming from the lips of a friend and fellow warrior can be overwhelming. Every aspect of law enforcement is designed towards ensuring your safety and the safety of those brothers and sisters serving alongside you. As a young officer in the academy, you are instructed that when a fellow officer calls for help you drop everything. While in your field training the concept broadens with the reality being drilled into you that if you hear those fateful words, an officer needs assistance, you move quicker, drive faster, and think of nothing other than getting there to help. I remember my field training officer, Mike Lacoss saying, "if you hear that an officer needs help you must drive by the seat of your pants, faster than you feel possible, pushing every limit both physically and mechanically to get there".

I never really understood exactly what he was implying because at one point he said I couldn't help if I didn't arrive safely, as it pertained to tactical driving, but now he was saying push the limits of not only myself but my vehicle. It wasn't until I heard my first, Officer needs Assistance call, that it all made sense. Through the radio the fear plagued voice of a fellow officer, alone in the dark, fighting for his life, pleading for help awoke a feeling inside which I can honestly say I hoped to never feel again. Although different in context, the officer standing before us, reaching the point where the stress and trauma has begun affecting him or her, is frightfully similar and should elicit the exact same response.

I can look in the mirror with pride that the men and women serving under me as their Sheriff felt confident enough in my compassion to seek help from me rather than fearing reprisal and keeping their pain inside. Whether it is the officer experiencing nightmares from a shooting, recurring thoughts from childhood trauma, or marital problems, police administrators must create a safe space where their people feel able to approach and seek out help. As we have discussed previously and will go in depth in the upcoming chapters of this offering, there is a wide array of possible coping mechanisms we can put into place to assist our officers and ourselves as we struggle to deal with trauma, depression, anxiety and overall stress.

Understandably, professional therapy is one of the most conventional means by which we can gain help. So, what is therapy all about? To answer this question, I felt the best answer would come from a therapist themself, so I approached a friend within the field. My friend, when asked what therapy was all about, simply said "it's a unbiased person who does their best to help people with trauma and unresolved issues through discussing effective ways to cope". In a nutshell, whether we research the topic in volumes of medical books, research papers, scholarly documents, or simply approach a friend, that's what therapy is all about.

For some people, officers included, engaging in therapy or professional counseling has helped them immensely. My friend and fellow officer Christian Martin described "both during and after I took part in therapy, I found that for the first time in my life I was able to connect the dots all the way back to my childhood. I was able to recognize how certain patterns and behaviors laid the foundation for the decisions I was making in my personal life." Like Christian, I have observed countless individuals who have struggled greatly with a wide array of trauma related stressors. Some struggled with addiction, some simply to look you in the eyes. I've stood by while officers who I have spoken to reluctantly begin the process of therapy, skeptical about the potential results only to come to me later describing how "it is really helping me".

For me, there is really no better feeling than seeing a person you have tried and tried to get help for finally break down and agree and then later smile with excitement as the doors to a bright future seemingly becomes available for them. Does it always happen this way, with excitement, and a renewed vision? No, but when we truly hope to engage our inner struggles, professional therapy can be a huge contributing factor for our success. Many wonder what therapy is all about and how it can possibly help. Those questions are valid and must be elaborated upon if we hope to help others.

The potential benefits to engaging in therapy are numerous including helping officers develop new coping mechanisms, enhancing deductive reasoning, providing insight, exploring the mind and enhancing self-development. In the end, the reason a person chooses to go to therapy may vary. Some people choose to engage a professional counselor because they are interested in doing better and personally growing. Others may choose to go to therapy because the things in their lives, relationships, or professional lives are becoming unbearable and simply said... something must give. When describing the reasons cops seek out the assistance of a professional counselor, Dr. Ellen Kirschman, a writer for psychology today writes "What may motivate you to ramp up the courage to seek help? Sometimes it's, emotional pain, rumination (non-stop negative thinking), Poor self-esteem, anxiety, high stress, grief, addictions, or self-destructive behavior".

As described earlier, there are several benefits to engaging with a professional counselor. Even if the only benefit is that we walk away from the sessions with a broader understanding of ways of coping with trauma and stress. Committing to visit a therapist can many times help us analyze why we have adapted to trauma in certain ways and explore whether our adaptations are truly helping us or not. The inclusion of a professional therapist can assist us as we look at changing the hard-formed habits we have learned over the years.

I often wondered what therapy was truly like. Would it be like the counselor depicted on the television, wearing a wrinkly coat, smoking a pipe, listening as I laid on a plaid-colored couch straight out of the 1970's? Or would it be something different? I have learned over the years, what I was seeing on television was not the reality of professional counseling. I've watched counselors engage their clients in a wide array of settings, some outside under a tree, and some in a traditional office space. Onah Caleb (2020) describes "Therapeutic sessions are done in a serene and peaceful environment where individuals do not feel guilty or insecure." She went on to describe "In a meeting, a therapist may not always tell individuals all they need to do but they try to assert thought processes from what is being said and those not through guidance".

In a nutshell, therapy assists us through pushing us outside our normal and comfortable environment in hopes that a new perspective will prove beneficial as we face the challenges we often face. Understanding the possible benefits to obtaining therapy, why then are so many officers hesitant to take the step? Simply said, officers many times have a difficult time trusting the process. One officer described it this way "I have not yet found a mental health professional that I feel completely comfortable talking to". What many fail to understand is that although great individuals and highly competent professionals, not all therapists can gain the trust of the law enforcement officer. Many times, officers need someone that understands their plight and truly "gets them" to fully find the benefit of therapy. Describing the rigors of police work to an empathetic soul who has never slept in a ditch, eaten up by ticks, felt hungry, or tired, or scared can be a daunting task.

I have heard it more times than I hoped to, officers describing behavioral health professionals as, well intentioned, caring people who the officer truly likes, but "they just don't get us". I liken it to the first youth group I led, as a youth pastor, in Colorado. While discussing fellow youth workers I had a small group of girls tell me that the other workers don't truly love them (the kids). Shocked, I inquired why the kids felt that way. My reasoning was because I felt I had a good grasp on my workers and the kid's comment was the furthest from the truth. The students explained that my wife and I spent time with the kids, the others only helped once a week and really didn't sacrifice any time with them to truly understand and know them. They went on to describe that they knew my wife and I loved them because we took the time to be with them.

Wow, what a slap in the face right? Similarly, trying to convince a officer that someone who has never experienced their struggles, or felt their pain, can help them through the pain is impossible even though an error. One officer from Colorado, as he described his experiences with professional counseling put it this way.

I tried counseling once about halfway through my career. It was a joke. Afterward I told myself never again. The counselor spent the first fifteen minutes covering the payment plan, which was a non-issue because the counseling was through my employee assistance program offered through my agency. I quickly realized that there were keywords that would have been reported back to my agency; suicide, depression, ect. Saying any of those words would have, I felt, put me on the radar with my command staff, and after seeing an officer lose his career over something similar, there was no way this counselor was getting any info out of me. In a nutshell, there was zero trust in that counselor, zero trust in the system.

The counseling I eventually searched for much later on was someone I vetted. I ensured I could first, trust and secondly someone who understood police work and thirdly, does this person care and can I resonate with the counselor. Finding the person who met those criteria made the world of difference.

Luckily, many areas throughout our country have begun to realize that our law enforcement officers, firefighters, and first responders require more than just a seat in the chair when considering professional therapy. It is essential, not unlike working with veterans, for success to truly be felt and lives impacted. The therapist or counselor must have a tie to the law enforcement community and an ability to understand their plight through experience. States such as Missouri have proactively addressed this issue through developing a First Responder Network of professional counselors who because of their background specialize in working with law enforcement officers. After being highly vetted, the professionals name is attached to a Crisis Intervention web site where officers can seek out a therapist who "gets them".

I found this aspect helpful. One of the proactive steps I took shortly after several of my officers were ambushed during a routine eviction call was, I required each of my staff members, not in the hospital, to attend one mandatory therapy session. I sprang into action and contacted my local community behavioral health liaison and within days he had five licensed counselors, set up at a local church for sessions. Feeling that I really didn't need the therapy myself, I committed to my troops and their health by making the decision that if I was making them attend, I too would attend. As I began my session with the counselor, I was somewhat skeptical because I didn't need any help, this was all about my people and my leadership. At least that's what I told myself. The counselor approached the session superbly. Beginning with a brief bio, the man described his military service and commitment to his field. The mere act of this man's taking the time to tell me about himself caused me to lower my proverbial walls of defense because "he got me", and in my mind he could understand me due to his military service.

The reason a person chooses to engage in professional therapy or not is many times highly personal. As described, therapy has proven highly effective for many law enforcement officers and non-law enforcement personnel. For some, the thought of sitting down and sharing one's feelings with a perfect stranger is outside the realm of possibility so other strategies to enhance our coping with stress is needed. Many have found value in a wide array of non-traditional coping measures.

Chapter Summary and Key Takeaways

- An officer asking for help with their emotions and mental health should be approached no differently than the officer on the street requesting emergency assistance.

·   Professional Therapy is the most conventional means for receiving proactive coping strategies.

·   Therapy, in its pure definition is an un-bias person who is attempting to help resolve trauma through teaching coping skills.

·   Therapy includes developing coping mechanisms, enhancing deductive reasoning, providing insight, and improving self-development.

·   For many law enforcement officers, finding a therapist who has been involved in law enforcement work or the military is essential because the therapist can understand the officer's plight better.

Chapter Eleven

Group / Peer Counseling

"A true friend is someone who sees the pain in your eyes while everyone else believes the smile on your face."

~Unknown

The power of compassion is incomparable. Many times, the simple act of reaching out to our brothers and sisters behind the badge with only the intent to lift them up lays the foundation for their recovery. I remember several years ago sitting along the front range in Colorado as a large flock of Canadian geese flew over- head. Their beauty was unquestionable and the grace with which they flew across the sky amazed me. I saw a similar sight recently as I traveled with my family to eastern Missouri for a scheduled appointment.

On this trip, rather than Canadian geese my girls and I had the opportunity to watch as a large gathering of snow geese graced us with their presence. The flock gently flowed in formation, perfectly spaced, until they found a resting place in a farm field beside the highway. As I described to my children what we were watching one of the girls asked, "why are they making that noise?" As the child made this statement, I could hear the audible sound of the geese "honking" to each other, some in unison, and others seemingly all alone.

The sound of the geese "honking" not only reminded me of my childhood, when as I watched the flock, I became entranced by the sounds the geese were making but it also caused me to smile. I remember sitting in church one Sunday, shortly after my first encounter with the geese when the pastor asked his congregation if they noticed the geese fly overhead. Excitingly, I raised my hand in agreement and shook my head, assuring him that I for one had observed it. What the pastor then described has stuck with me over the years. He began telling the congregation that when flocks of geese are traveling, they have a unique behavior which not only allows them to maintain course and a sense of direction but likewise it provides encouragement to one another.

The pastor described that the honking which we hear is that behavior. He spoke about how we often hear the geese in the back "honk away" seemingly encouraging the birds in the front to maintain their course and continue onward. Describing when its time to flap their wings and when it's alright to glide. Remembering that story, I quickly imparted the fun fact to my own children. As I have grown, I have often thought about the "honking" of the geese and how truly genius the concept is. A concept so rich in possibility if we are only committed enough to put it to use. I have come accustomed to referring to the concept as "honk therapy". Who couldn't benefit from this form of a little therapy?

As humans, there is little difference when we consider the benefit of honking to one another as a form of encouragement. Mankind it seems, especially in these modern times, thrive contact and reassuring interaction. Who doesn't like it when a friend or even stranger tells us we are doing good or looking great. My youngest child Riyann has this concept down to a tee. Her mother and I began noticing that the child routinely sought out strangers anytime we were in public. As any red-blooded parent can attest, this scared us to death. The time-honored principle of stranger danger simply hadn't taken hold in Riyann's mind.

With each contact, Riyann would either engage strangers in conversation or in many cases walk up to them, give them a big hug, and retreat back to us. I remember one day, as we walked into the grocery store, she noticed an elderly lady walking out of the store. Leaving my side, Riyann approached the woman and began engaging her in conversation, "your hair looks beautiful today and I really like the scarf you are wearing" Riyann stated. The woman, taken back, but quickly smiled and described how thankful she was to the little girl. Returning to my side, a smile affixed to her face, we continued our journey. When we got back in the car to leave, I asked her why she said that to the stranger. Her response was the kind of response which warms one's heart. Riyann described that the woman looked like she was having a hard day and she hoped that by showing a little kindness, the woman's day would be brighter. Taking the role of the geese, the child simply "honked" away in hopes that her words impacted another's life.

Whether it is the "honking" of the geese or the kind words and actions of a little eight-year- old girl, we can find a significant example of encouragement. As Officers struggle with trauma and the effects the trauma is having on them personally, many disregard the importance of simple encouragement. Many times, a kind gesture, warm hug, or even a non-critical listening ear can have major impact on struggling individuals. One manner by which the law enforcement community has begun addressing trauma and the overall wellness and resiliency of their officers is through the use of peer groups or peer counseling.

As we noted earlier, many law enforcement officers struggle with traditional means of coping because of a reluctance to engage professionals with little to no experience in the way law enforcement officers act or think. Providing them with another option has proven successful in many instances. As Emily Cnapich describes (2022) "There is an overwhelming need to manage the mental health and psychological well-being of emergency service workers. To address these concerns, peer support programs have garnered increased interest and support from the first responder community".

Understanding that police officers have a unique yet stressful job, it is easy to see the tough exterior, hardened actions, and strict adherence to guidelines but even easier to fail to see the internal struggles associated with the environment these men and woman serve within. With this in mind, one could easily understand why officers may hesitate to speak to doctors, psychologists, or clergy but would welcome speaking to another police officer. Why is this? Simply said, again, other officers understand them. Some may wonder why I keep beating this concept into your mind, again and again... Simply said, it is that important. Firmly grasping what it's going to take to help these officers will cause us to do the exact same thing we are asking them to do. We must exit our perceived comfort zone of beliefs and stigma and enter their realm.

The inclusion of options outside the traditional method of meeting the needs of those suffering from unresolved trauma, primarily therapy, is not only essential but likewise welcome within the law enforcement community. As described by Coon (2018) "Peer support members are there to provide guidance and support to fellow officers...during any kind of distressing situation". As many departments throughout the United States buy into the peer support concept, teams are being trained and compiled to meet the needs of our officers.

Routinely undergoing a basic series of crisis intervention training, peer support team members are uniquely equipped to be activated in a wide array of situations where officers or groups of officers are affected. Having real life experience aids these officers as they interact with their peers and further the mission of providing pertinent, confidential assistance in the officer's time of need. One of the present misconceptions within the realm of peer support is that the trained peer support officers must have experienced the same gravity of trauma the officer has to be effective. This is errant. In reality, some officers may have lived through similar situations, that's a plus, but in the end, experiencing similar crisis related incidents and merely walking the same streets, working the same shifts, experiencing the career as a whole, aids the officers with providing relevant assistance to their brothers and sisters.

This is why many times a military veteran can be an effective therapist or peer worker to our law enforcement officers. Although differing in many aspects, the similarities between law enforcement and the military afford a sense of comradery. Both have worked long hours, under adverse conditions, been asked to perform tasks which the common man would hesitate and followed similar hierarchies. Many others overlook the human aspect of our law enforcement officers and simply view the need along with its association to job related stressors.

Bearing similar importance, peer trained support personnel are uniquely poised to provide encouragement and strategies relating to non- work-related stressors such as relational, financial, and health related situations which may arise. Although peer team members are routinely fellow officers, an important aspect to the program is a collaboration with other trained and licensed behavioral health professionals in the event that a peer welcomes a referral for more detailed behavioral health treatment. Additionally, the inclusion among the peer teams or peer group trainers of supervisory personnel is rare and for the most part avoided.

The reasoning behind this is an officer has to feel a certain level of comfort confronting his or her perceived weak points and struggles and speaking to a supervisor can many times be frowned upon. The fact that the supervisor is more than likely a good listener and confidant means little. The overwhelming fear of reprisal and worse paves the path of avoidance and must be considered if we truly want to effect change. Being a law enforcement administrator myself, this is an area I had to deal with. Although well intentioned I had to learn that some of my troops simply wouldn't approach me with certain problems.

The reluctance on part of my guys didn't stem from a mistrust but simply a reasonable fear. No-one wants to tell the boss they are feeling vulnerable. You won't find any officer who truly wants his or her boss to see them in that light. Although in most cases the furthest from the truth, the risk is just too great. Hence, peer group counselors are routinely not of the supervisory group.

One of the common statements I said to teenagers I had encountered while working the streets, who were struggling, was that they needed to find a trusted adult that they and their family trusted. Saying this I would quickly be met with questioning eyes from parents and confusion from the kids. I would often expound on my statement by describing that having a trusted adult to run things by, confide in, and share with, many times helped them gain a new perspective on age old problems. The main reason I would attempt to share this truth with younger citizens is my knowledge that regardless of how strong the parent child bond was, there was a reluctance to tell mom and dad certain things. Why? Because we don't want to disappoint them. Think about it, would a teenage girl, deeply in love, feel comfortable speaking to her highly religious parents about safe sexual activity? Would a young man who has been told to avoid a certain friend because of some sense that trouble is brewing, feel comfortable relaying to his dad that he was at a party the night before with the boy? No, in both cases most likely. It isn't because the child doesn't care for or trust their parents but, in their minds, there are just some things they don't want to tell. Each time I shared this concept with a new child, my words were always met with a shaking of the head in agreement.

The same rings true for adults. Officers simply avoid telling supervisors some things which they feel are too personal or could possibly depict them in a negative light. Likewise, peer group members are rarely licensed counselors. Although receiving specialized training as described, they are simply brothers and sisters there to ensure your needs are met and that you are aware of every resource available.

Unlike the honking of the geese, the trained brother or sisters in law enforcement who knows best what you are going through, understands. Officers who have a brother or sister available to call and just say "hey, got a second to talk?" will be able to feel a greater level of support and know that people have their six. The selfless actions of peer team members create confidence within the department and in the end make it easier to solicit help from professionals if required.

The inclusion of peer teams associated with law enforcement mental health paves the path for success. As described, some officers can and will benefit from formal therapy while others simply refuse to even consider the possibility. Does this mean the officer is destined for a future filled with pain and suffering? No, along with the conventional mechanisms of coping like therapy and peer group counseling, several other non-conventional modes of coping exists which if applied can assist our law enforcement partners successfully overcome the demons of the calling.

Chapter Summary and Key Takeaways

·   Humans can observe a great example of effective interaction from the common goose. Coined as "Honk Therapy" the mere act of encouraging one another can not only improve our outlook but likewise keep us on the right path.

·   Peer counseling, although not conducted by licensed therapist, is a avenue by which peers with similar experience and training can effectively "understand" and guide others.

·   Having similar experiences often aids with counseling and understanding and creates a more effective means by which positive outcomes can be experienced.

·   To avoid any hesitation or concerns over retaliation, supervisory personnel should avoid actively taking on the role of peer counselor.

Chapter Twelve

Non-Conventional Methods

"The scariest moment is always just before you start."

~Stephen King

My life, regardless of which moment I was embroiled in, seldom followed the strict series of conventional stereotypes set forth by history or society. Whether it was my time in the Navy, serving as a mayor, or working alongside my brothers and sisters, fighting evil upon the streets of America, my path was simply my own. It wasn't that I shunned normality, I in fact preached a sense of conformity. Rather, I always seemed to be confronted by unique situations and hence had to travel the paths of life in my own way. One aspect I am genuinely proud about is the fact that regardless of what I was confronted by, I always attempted to see the good, and make the best of any given situation to ensure that I came out sparkly clean on the other side.

For many officers, the conventional manners by which we find assistance when dealing with the trauma and stressors associated with our chosen field are simply out of reach. Some fear the unknown aspects of seeking help while others refuse to lower their defense shields, trusting another with their innermost secrets. As we discussed earlier, many officers don't feel there is even an issue because everything they are experiencing is just part of the job. Many fall under the same or similar belief systems as I did which leaves them seeing minimal rewards for speaking up or stepping onto the ledge.

At what point my worldview was established is uncertain. I like to think that it was in fact a result of a lifetime of learning and experience. For me, recognizing that the stress and trauma was potentially getting to me was more than just a choice. I had conditioned myself, over the years, to avoid the feelings of stress and trauma and to replace them with other thoughts, good thoughts about adventure, people, and opportunities. For me, to dwell on the bad gave it a place at the proverbial table.

I was asked recently what I meant when I say, "giving it a place at the table". In my mind, and in my own special way, the only truly valuable answer to that question could come from a personal example. Although I will not get into particulars, the story I will share will give you a better insight into my idea of giving our problems a seat at the table.

As a child, I was truly blessed. Although far from rich in the monetary sense, my family's wealth was instead distributed through love and experience. My parents provided for all their children's needs while maintaining a strict adherence to the rules of the house. The times were just different in the mid to late seventies. What parents allowed their children to do would be seen as crazy in modern times. I adventured most of my days, seldom worrying about anything or anyone. I knew to avoid the house down the street which had been widely known as the "hippie" house and other than staying out of trouble, my days were filled with learning from the hard knocks that life tends to supply.

My first experience with trauma was when I was around eleven or so and stemmed from a situation I, nor my family had expected nor would have ever envisioned. Without getting into particulars, I will just say the confusion and embarrassment which resulted would not only shape my immediate future but likewise prove foundational to the establishment of my worldview today. Looking back, I could have easily become a victim and forever assigned a feeling of dismay and dirtiness to my existence. Instead, I moved forward and refused to allow the event to become an established part of my mind or life. I didn't allow what happened to me to have a seat at the table per se.

My father always said, those who are seated at the dinner table are special. Whether family, friend, or guest, if we allow them to be seated, we must revere their position at the table and provide them with a place in our lives. The concept can transition to not only the dinner table but be inclusive of any table we are at. The conference table, strategy table, or church table, all bear the same significance. For me, recognizing and dwelling upon the trauma of life gives it a seat at the table of my heart and mind, hence forever giving it credence. I was committed young to avoid this line of thinking and to not fall victim to the "victim mentality".

In a way, that one event shaped every aspect of my life today. I still think about my decision to not succumb to being a victim. Each time I interviewed a victim of certain crimes I secretly hoped that they would be able to get the help necessary, to ensure that the event didn't overtake their future. Likewise, I had to catch myself when I was confronted by someone who had a firmly established "victim's mentality" and had become accustomed to blaming every aspect of their lives on a singular incident. or heard someone. Understanding that what they went through or had experienced is highly personal, I fought back the urge to be un-empathetic and bit my lip to ensure I didn't direct them to "get over it" and "move on". For me it was easy, for others it may not be so.

This concept of being easy for some and difficult to others is directly relative to the aspect of the overall wellness and resiliency of our men and woman in public service. The mere fact of what or how we choose to deal with the stressors in our lives can stem from events, education, or worldviews, we have learned over the years. Luckily, the options available for a public servant to seek and receive help vary significantly. In our modern times, failure to address our overall wellness is truly a choice in my opinion. Over the next several chapters of this offering, we will explore several non-conventional coping mechanisms designed to effectively counter the damage of stress and trauma while enhancing our overall resiliency.

The textbook definition of non-conventional is "not conventional: not conforming to convention, custom, tradition, or usual practice" (Webster, 2022). For many years, I failed to realize the need for countermeasures in my own life. As described, I had it all under control and my focus was on the welfare of my pack, or team. If I began feeling a buildup of stress, I simply willed myself out of it. It worked for me. I would quickly recover and be on my way, doing what I did best, serving my community. What I didn't realize is that I hadn't "willed myself" out of anything. I simply pushed my stressors to the back burner of my mind, shoving it really far back.

What I came to realize, as time flew by was the mere act of shoving my stress and trauma back, deep in my mind would expose me to behaviors which would surface at the spur of the moment, affecting my moods, outlooks, and demeanor. A prime example of this was when my beautiful wife and I had the opportunity to represent our county in Washington D.C. while visiting the white house. Our excitement was heightened and the thought of meeting the President of the United States brought an immensely proud yet nervous feeling over both of us. I remember the second day was set aside when we could take a moment and explore our nation's capital and all the historic sites. We had arranged the perfect tour. As we prepared to get on the tour bus, I found my seat and while looking to my wife, it seemed neither of us could contain our excitement.

As the tour bus began to move, I briefly looked at my cellular telephone, preparing to ensure that everything was in order for what would prove to be a day filled with picture taking to document our adventure. What I saw next changed my entire outlook, thrusting me into a heightened level of stress. As I opened my phone, I noticed the battery level was very low. Although connected to the charger, or at least I thought it was connected, my phone had failed to charge from the night before. For what should have been a miniscule problem I immediately transitioned into a heightened state of stress.

I could feel the cold sweat coming on and the anxiety rise. As I mentioned to my wife, hoping she had a charger in her purse, the thoughts of no one being able to contact me if needed compounded my anxiety. Disregarding the fact that I was thousands of miles away from home, and how truly could I help anyone calling the good ol sheriff for help, I remained in a state of overload. It wasn't until my wife, and I made the next stop at the Mall of America, purchased a battery pack at a exorbitant cost, and took a half hour to charge my phone that I found solace.

For something so miniscule as a poorly charged battery to totally affect my outlook was astounding. For the event to affect my stress and ultimate health was more so concerning. In my mind, it wasn't simply the cellular telephone's battery level which caused the reaction but in truth, the flowing over of all the stress I kept ineffectively dealing with. My emotions surfaced, seemingly using the battery as a medium for a much deeper issue.

Ensuring that one doesn't succumb to the overflowing of emotion due to unresolved stress and trauma can be accomplished through a wide variety of conventional and unconventional means. For me, to truly feel the positive affect of successfully coping with my stress, I had to take proactive steps to ensure that I not only dealt with the issues but likewise that I was able to recognize the need for effectively coping in spite of my warrior-based mentality of strength and endurance through any challenge.

Being uniquely different, each person must find what works best for them when considering the most effective way to cope with stress and trauma. For some, talking to others or talking to a professional counselor is all it takes. For many others, that's just not their cup of tea and nonconventional coping strategies such as writing, exercise, and the faith factor are essential modes of survival. Regardless, we have an obligation to act. An obligation not only to ourselves to find the solution but an obligation to our loved ones and families. For it is within the eyes of our children that we find hope and they find the way.

Chapter Summary and Key Takeaways

·   The ease of decision making as it relates to our behavioral health is multifaceted and is dependent on many factors such as timing, personal worldviews, and overall resilience.

·   Failure to implement effective coping strategies in one's life can lead to momentary over stimulation of emotions, rendering us unable to deal with minor issues which can arise.

·   Non-conventional means of enhancing resilience and coping with stress, although differing in content, can provide a platform for effective coping strategies and overall wellness.

·   Being uniquely different, one person may find certain coping mechanisms effective while others fail to find significance in the manner chosen. In the end, it is each of our responsibilities to find what works for them as they struggle with trauma and stress.

·   Finding the most effective coping strategy is a truly personal thing. The inclusion of both traditional and non-conventional manners to cope should be explored.

Chapter Thirteen

Writing/ Journaling

"Nothing will work unless you do."

~Maya Angelou

Writing, to me, was always a concept which bore little significance. I remember as my father aged, he and I had gotten into the habit of getting together on Saturday mornings. We would meet at the local diner and enjoy a breakfast, just two men, discussing everything from how unreasonable people were and the world as we knew it. Although usually only a couple hours in duration, the weekly get together became something I not only loved but needed. During one of those meals, I remember my dad describing how proud he was of me. I had recently been elected to the position of Mayor in the city we lived in. The act of being elected was a feat, when you really think about it. For a middle-aged, divorced man coupled with the fact I was considered an outsider, to be elected was a thing no one saw coming.

In addition to my age, marital status, and residency, the fact that I truly never placed much emphasis on anything other than law enforcement ended up causing some to wonder what the future held for our little town. I remember dad asking me several months prior to the election why I wanted to run for office. The answer somewhat eluded me. Sure, things were happening in the small, rural town in Missouri that I disagreed with and sure I felt I could affect some positive change, especially where the town's law enforcement was concerned. But the truth behind my candidacy was much simpler than that.

It all began with a simple trip to the grocery store. While shopping, I remember being approached by an elderly resident. Smiling, she introduced herself and told me she had heard me speak at one of the previous city council meetings. As we spoke, she grabbed my arm with hers and said "son, we need you to run for Mayor". Smiling, I maintained my silence. I had never filled that type of role and to be honest never had a desire to. Being ever hesitant to disappoint people and having a soft spot in my heart for older ladies, her persistence paid off and I told her I would think long and hard about it. Unfortunately for me this answer wasn't good enough and she refused to relent until I agreed to run for office. Telling dad, the true story of my candidacy resulted in a slight grin. The kind of grin only dad could do, which sent the message that I had no worldly idea of what was to come.

As dad and I spoke, he began elaborating on why he was so proud of me. He described that he recalled two instances when I was in school. The first was in the fifth grade when he was approached by my teacher. My teacher, he said, had told him that he had great concerns for me because I simply couldn't learn the content he was teaching. He told dad he felt I needed to be moved to a special education area of the school. Knowing me better than anyone, dad simply explained that my difficulty learning was not stemming from a learning difficulty but rather a problem with laziness.

The second instance dad spoke of was during my senior year in high school where dad met with my guidance counselor. He described that this kind woman had told him that she was genuinely concerned about me. She added that her concern was over my inability to communicate effectively with others. Not unlike my previous teacher, dad simply reassured her that I would be fine and all it was going to take was for me to find my place in this world. As my father relayed these two stories to me, we laughed, although I must admit, my interest was piqued. "You proved them all wrong son" he said with a smile. "Look where you are now". Little did dad know that within five years not only would his son be a mayor and highly respected figure in the state, but also the sheriff in the county dad grew up in, speaking with people dad only dreamed of meeting and traveling to places many find impossible. All because I was blessed with a dad who refused to accept mediocrity and had his son's back at all costs.

The fact that I had at least two educators who voiced concern over my education was not a surprise to me. As I said earlier, when I attended grade, middle and high school my motivation was far from schoolwork. It seemed girls and sports were truly all I really cared about. The problem was, I definitely was not a ladies' man. My awkward, somewhat goofy self didn't have the impact on the girls I had hoped for so for the most part I was destined to thrive along the sports front. Even in adulthood, I never gave much thought to the act of writing. Sure, work required certain reports to be in the written form so I would get by, effectively, but that's where my writing ended.

While I was a Sheriff in Carter County Missouri, I began finding my place as a person who could effectively communicate in the written form. With each newspaper article I wrote I found more and more enjoyment. The accolades from readers added to my thought that I may be a decent writer, so I became more and more motivated to place my thoughts to paper. I always found calmness with writing down my thoughts. For just a moment, I could remove myself from my surroundings and lay out plans to help our community and all those in it. With each article written, I became embolden.

It wasn't until I sat at home, watching a news report about the Ferguson Missouri protests that I began considering writing on a larger scale. What I saw on the television angered me, to be quite honest. Regardless of if the actions of the officer were rational and lawful, what I was seeing was a complete distortion of truth. I watched as the media, leaders, and even the President of the United States portrayed all law enforcement officers as "bad" and in need of a radical overhaul. My anger turned to action as I penned a news article. The article encompassed the true depiction of those serving their communities. Not feeling that I truly got my word across I decided at that time to write a book.

My hope was that through this book, The Calling, the reader could truly get a glimpse into what it is to be an officer in America today. I would allow each reader into the mind of our officers, what motivates them, what makes them tick, their fears, desires, and dreams. What I had never imagined was that the mere act of beginning the writing process would in fact become a majorly therapeutic and soul revealing experience for me. With each word, I found relief. With each sentence I was able to expose my own truth, reservations, and struggles. With each page, I exposed my innermost fears and pain.

Although difficult at times, the mere act of being highly personal with the understanding that others, some known to me and some unknown, would read my words proved both overwhelming and yet eerily satisfying. In the end, as I penned the final words, a strong sense of accomplishment flowed over me. It seemed that each time I described an event or incident which caused me pain, the feelings of grief and angst were erased for a time. It's difficult to explain, but for me, writing became my basis for coping.

Countless others, some inside the law enforcement works and others not, have found writing to be an effective coping strategy when dealing with stress and trauma. One officer, describing the benefits he received from taking the time to write down his thoughts in a journal said, "I began to journal, it was an eye opener to me." He added "Journaling helped me identify patterns in my life". The act of journaling or writing is not unlike some of us who kept a diary or journal when we were children.

Think back to when you were younger. If you kept a diary, how did it make you feel? As described in the University of Rochester Medical Center encyclopedia (2023) "you might have kept a diary under your mattress when you were a teenager. It was a place to confess your struggles and fears without judgment or punishment. It likely made you feel good to write down your thoughts." The author goes on to describe "the world seemed clearer." Although many who used a diary when they were younger discontinued its use in adulthood, the concept and benefits remain.

One of the main ways to deal with stress and trauma is to establish a healthy manner by which we can learn to deal with our emotions. The modern-day diary, a journal or journaling is just that. Many have found that the simple act of writing down their thoughts in a journal is an effective way to cope. The University of Rochester goes on to described that the benefits of writing or journaling include helping to manage anxiety, reduce stress, and coping with depression. Some of the countless benefits of writing or journaling include the facts that when journaling a person is better equipped to recognize and prioritize problems, fears, and concerns while providing a unique opportunity to identify contributing factors and engage in self-help mechanisms.

As for me, writing can many times help identify what is causing stress and in turn help me establish a plan to conquer the issue through positive resolution processes. Jon Reed (2022), content writer for Publishing Talk describes "from clearer thinking to greater confidence that comes from mastering a skill to processing difficult life events there are plenty of ways writing can give you a boost." Reed continued by describing that writing allows one to think clearer because the mere process includes the importance of clearly defining what you hope to portray. Additionally, the process of writing allows you to more effectively process emotions and experiences.

Research, according to Reed (2022) shows that writing about what "hurts" or causes us pain can ultimately improve our mental health. In addition to the benefits of broadening our coping mechanisms, writing can many times increase our self-awareness and inner happiness. In the end, if it makes you happy to write, it is something we can benefit from.

Will writing erase any need for professional counseling or therapy in the present or future? Most likely not. But what journaling can do is provide a means by which a person can effectively engage a coping strategy which can lessen the effects of stress and trauma while at times identifying the reason behind our anxiety. For me, the mere act of putting my word to paper did just that. I felt my anxiety leave like clockwork as I dove into my writing and exploration.

One potential drawback to writing in the manner which I chose, the book form, is that it becomes a bearing of one's soul. A book is public where a journal is highly private. Although the act of writing my book was refreshing, I was allowing others in and that could prove uncomfortable, especially given the typical responses from my brothers and sisters in blue. As I completed my first book, although feeling accomplished and hopeful that others will finally understand if they approached the subject with an open mind. I laid out my innermost experiences and feelings for the world to see.

Would the second goal of my writing, the hope that officers will gain a better understanding of wellness? Had I accomplished that too or would they simply consider me weak? This was a challenge for me. But in the end the benefits of telling my story won out and although my fears persist, they are slowly being overcome with each message, telephone call and physical contact I have with officers thanking me for telling my story and helping them. In the end, writing became the crux for this once considered illiterate man to cope and broaden the understanding of stress and trauma for countless others.

Chapter Summary and Key Takeaways

· Writing or journaling can prove to be an effective tool when coping with stress and anxiety.

· The mere act of writing down one's problems, experiences, and stressors opens the door to recognizing root causes and effects.

· Writing cannot assure you that therapy or other conventional manners of coping will not be needed and should be used as a tool.

· Writing can be extremely personal, and exposure can bring out new anxieties and stress if not addressed adequately.

Chapter Fourteen

Health / Fitness

"All progress takes place outside the comfort zone."
~ Michael John Bobak

B eing young and full of energy, I seldom gave much thought to the benefits of a stringent health and fitness routine. I was confident in my ability to perform, and when it mattered, I could easily bolster the energy necessary to overcome any obstacle. I was unable to draw an inference between physical health and mental health because to be quite candid, It never seemed important. Sure, I fully understood the benefits to increasing my endurance as well as making sure my strength was adequate to win any physical struggle, I was involved in. Understanding that there is a direct correlation between physical health and mental health didn't come until much later in life.

The aspect of fitness, and the need to maintain it, became apparent to me the first time I dawned the protective defensive tactics suit. Covering every portion of my body, the red pads in a sense made me feel invincible. I would be able to sustain a strike, hit, or kick without feeling the impact, all while vehemently attacking the students in an attempt to teach them the importance of proper tactics.

As a young defensive tactic's instructor, I had prepped my students for real life situations. It was now the time to put their training and commitment to the test. Each student would get the opportunity to fight me, one on one, using anything at their disposal as long as it wasn't lethal or taser related for three minutes. As I conspired with my co-instructor, the radiant feeling of excitement filled the room. For me, I was going to show these kids how the big boy's roll. For the students, this was their opportunity to reciprocate the pain their instructors had been administering the entire week. As the starting bell rang, the fight was on and through laughter, audible grunts and groans, and a great deal of shuffling around, I was able to maintain my footing and survive my first student encounter.

As the second simulation began, I immediately felt the weight of the burdensome protective suit. As the sweat began to dribble down every orifice of my body, I began feeling weary. With each attack my energy depleted more and more leaving me with one goal in mind, the goal of survival. Although exhausted, a good instructor never lets their students see them struggling. While taking an opportune break, a command decision was made to switch out instructors between each student to allow us "big boys" to catch a breather.

Although preaching about stamina to our students was a constant for both me and my fellow instructors, the reality was that our own stamina wasn't really all that good. To be quite honest with you, that wasn't going to change. Why wasn't it going to change? Simply put, we were young and for the most part it wasn't a priority in our minds. We could easily sidetrack the discussion, explaining that the reason we became so exhausted was due to the necessity of wearing a sixty-pound protective suit. When in reality, the suit had little to do with our stamina.

For many years, the illusion of infallibility and overall invincibility reigned supreme for me just as it has for countless others in my position. I had other, more important things to do than to waste countless hours in a gym, track, or ring, fine tuning my strength and endurance. If I needed to survive I would. If I was confronted by a combative situation, I could conjure up the energy to overcome and safely go home that night. Time was a commodity, and although wrong as it was, fitness and overall wellness was not a priority of the young Richard Stephens.

The illusion of time was reiterated by Michael C. Harper (2023) when he wrote "Quite often the lack of time is cited as a major reason not to exercise", as he described common barriers to fitness among law enforcement officers. Although it is widely known that the benefits of exercise supersede any negative ramifications, many officers simply do not place a priority in fitness. A shift in reasoning must take place to ensure overall wellness and resiliency.

As any seasoned officer can attest, the link between physical fitness and stress relief, or mental wellness exists whether we wish to admit it openly. Bradley Williams, Member of the Victoria Police and former Australian Army member describes (2018) "Studies suggest that regular exercise is one of the best things for helping manage stress". He goes on to state "when you exercise regularly, it gets endorphins flowing, which puts you in a good mood and helps you feel good about yourself". Studies have shown that a person's mental health is bolstered through fitness training on many levels including the most simplistic approach of simply taking the time away to place your mind on things other than what is bringing you stress.

When a person exercises, they in a sense are accomplishing multiple things simultaneously. First, they are helping their body become more fit and secondly, you do the same for your mind, helping it become more fit. In a field such as law enforcement, or first responder, we all know the job can and will be stressful. This is where the importance of ensuring your mind maintains a high level of fitness results in lasting benefits.

I can't disagree with the assertion that physical fitness is beneficial, we all know it is. Likewise, looking back on my journey, I am reminded of the many times I purchased the latest book on fitness, the most recent fad diet, and even began the process of going to the gym routinely. What I was never able to commit to was the long term follow through. Again, I never made it a priority. For me it was always a time factor. In reality, an excuse of time being the issue.

The experts say to fully benefit from an exercise and fitness routine; one should set aside thirty-minutes each day for physical activity. Due to the busy lifestyles of law enforcement, many find the possibility of their setting aside thirty-minutes for fitness impossible. Luckily, recent research has shown that "multiple, short bouts of exercise of at least ten minutes can also be effective". In the end, we can all find ten minutes each day if it is important to us. The key is determining just how imperative our fitness is.

In a perfect world, each of us would make our fitness a priority and respond as my good friend and brother Christian always has. My brother gets up each day and heads out on a four to five mile run before work. I remember his inviting me along on multiple occasions, an invitation I graciously denied, numerous times, describing that long runs simply weren't my thing. Looking back, my reluctance rarely involved my inability to try, or my desire to be better fit, but rather, my refusal to experience the initial pain of getting back into shape and the time it would entail.

The role of police officer or first responder is filled with emotion as we all know. Hypervigilance and critical incidents cause multiple stress hormones to be released into our blood stream in order to enhance our survivability. The problem is that later, those same hormones can impede our problem solving and complex reasoning portions of our brain. Additionally, the constant influx of stress induced hormones can, in layman's terms, add to the spare tire we often find around our mid-section as we age. When we exercise, we are helping our bodies rid ourselves of the stress induced hormones we are storing within our bodies. This allows us to think more clearly while experiencing "feel good" moments, allowing us to fend off depressive and anxiety rattled moments.

Nutrition also plays a key factor in not only our physical fitness but likewise our mental health. Like no other career, the law enforcement and first responder worlds are void any opportunity for a prolonged opportunity to sit and enjoy a meal hence it is very common for officers to resort to available fast-food restaurants. Being readily available and open for service twenty-four hours per day, food which touts convenience and lack substance become the norm for officers who rely on a quick, eat on the go convenience of fast food.

The problem therein is many times, the meals lack the adequate nutritional value necessary to sustain. Leaving officers and first responders to welcome the quick fix, of foods high in sugar content and with high carbohydrates. The high sugars, although let's face it, enjoyable, lead to weight gain, heart disease, and high cholesterol. How many times, after finishing up the latest value meal, have you been left with a tired, foggy feeling? For me, more times than I'd like to admit.

Failing to adequately ensure healthy eating habits many times lead to a deficiency in the body's necessary chemicals and minerals including B12, D3 and amino acids. As medical professionals can attest to when we lack the minimum levels of these crucial vitamins, we can experience a wide variety of negative reactions including brain fog, depression, memory loss, irritability, many times mimicking dementia. It has been proven that lower levels of D3 can also affect our body's muscle mass, leaving us many times with joint and muscle pain.

Engaging in healthy eating habits will have a lasting effect for officers striving to serve their communities. Generally, avoiding empty calories such as processed junk food, chips and candy is essential. Empty calories cause the human body to initially feel fulfilled but rapidly cause us to "crash" and feel lethargic. Additionally, empty calories encourage the body to store fat. One of the best examples I have seen to avoiding empty calories was written by George Vrotsos, writer for Police One. George described (2016) "You wouldn't put dirty fuel in your squad car, so don't put it into your body".

It is important that we eat nutrient-dense whole foods like real meats, vegetables, fruit, eggs, and nuts to not only fulfill our desire for food but also to meet our health-related needs. Easy enough, right? Wrong, in our fast-paced lives choosing the proper nutrient rich options can be a daunting task. Following the below listed guidelines, penned by

Police One, can assist us with ensuring that we are putting the best possible fuel into our bodies.

- When buying food on duty- choose the grilled option
- Try eating at a "make your own" taco/ burrito bar.
- Modify your fast food by ordering it wrapped in lettuce rather than a bun. Order fruit rather than fries.
- Prepare your own meal and take it to work with you.

In short, the time has long come that we truly take a look at our fitness and eating habits if we hope to maintain not only our physical wellbeing but likewise our mental resiliency. Not unlike changes in case and statutory law, we can complain about it, but we need to begin prioritizing our health. All of us can take an extra fifteen minutes each day to take a walk or ten minutes to do some activities designed to enhance our health. I remember a short time ago when my wife and I were talking about trying to eat healthier. My wife described that her goal was to live long enough to see our children grow up and get married. Continuing down the same path we were taking could not guarantee that end result and quite possibly sabotaged our plight. Instead, we would need to make sacrifices and do better to accomplish that goal.

Our lives as law enforcement officers are no different. We each start out with the goal of service. To be the savior and hero to those within the communities we serve. Whether we like it or not, regardless of if we agree with the premise or hate the very thought, prioritizing our health is a must to accomplish those goals. As we look at the unconventional ways of dealing with stress and trauma, health and fitness is crucial. As hard as it is to hear that, trust me it's more difficult to say it, understanding fully, that I must prioritize my health to sustain my own life.

Chapter Summary and Key Takeaways

- There is a direct correlation between physical activity and emotional/ mental health.
- Experts recommend thirty minutes of exercise daily. In the event time does not allow the recommended exercise multiple, ten-minute bouts of exercise has proved effective.
- Proper nutrition and exercise helps lower stress induced hormones in the body.
- We must all make fitness and nutrition a priority.

Chapter Fifteen

Mindset / Mindfulness

"The first and best victory is to conquer self."

~Plato

Shortly after my retirement from a thirty-year career in law enforcement I sat down at my new desk preparing for a virtual meeting. I had gone from a career field where most interactions were in person and very few meetings were instigated to a new career where meetings seemed to fill my days. The mere thought of attending a meeting virtually was somewhat foreign to me. In law enforcement everything was face to face until we experienced the COVID-19 pandemic. Due to enhanced concern and added fears of exposure many within the behavioral health community brainstormed and developed safe ways to carry out the goals of collaboration and safety, meeting online was the result.

My first few months within the behavioral health community was extremely informative as I learned that these people, my friends in behavioral health were truly the same species, of wolves, as my brothers and sisters in law enforcement although definitely not from the same pack. With shared goals and commitments, I could truly sense a kindship brewing and felt a sense of excitement over learning new and innovative ways to enhance the safety of my brothers and sisters in blue.

As I logged into the computer, I noticed a great deal of smiling faces and energy which peaked my attention. As I watched and listened, I found myself being drawn in. What I hadn't realized was that without warning the meeting would evolve into something I had never experienced and to be quite honest, left me shaking my head. We, in law enforcement, often joke about behavioral health and social type workers being "touchy feely" or "otherworld, sensitive" types who like to sit around getting in touch with their feelings. Behavioral attributes which for the most part is void in any down home, good-hearted, red-blooded cop. It made us feel weird, uncomfortable in a way. There I sat, sucked into my worst nightmare. I had entered one such meeting. A meeting where the proctor spoke about concentrating on our breathing, seeing our heartbeat, thinking about every part of our bodies, and envisioning the perfect scenery. I was left with only one option, that option was to mute my video so no one on the other end could see me shaking my head and lifting my jaw in amazement.

As I continued in the meeting, I couldn't bring myself to become engaged through participation in the wide array of mindfulness exercises they were teaching. I had a reputation to uphold, and we super cops simply didn't do these types of things. Flashing a welcoming smile, nodding every now and then and giving thanks was truly all I could muster. What had I gotten myself into? Was the remainder of my working life going to consist of hugging, smiles, and thoughts of pretty birds and ocean waves as this six-foot-seven beast of a man came to grips with his more sensitive side? All I knew at that moment was that I would have to go down fighting.

Over the next year and countless online meetings, even though I couldn't bring myself to participate very much, I found that I felt better. My stress was reduced, and I actually began welcoming the jovial spirit of my newly found friends. I learned that the mere act of surrounding yourself with positive thoughts and positive people added to my own enjoyment in life. Although, not fully convinced in the total breakdown in masculinity, in my opinion, of becoming engaged in the activities I was witnessing, the results were visible and beyond reproach. The act of concentrating or becoming mindful of my surroundings allowed me to lighten the burden I was feeling inside, becoming more focused on the positives in life.

When considering mindfulness as it relates to reducing stress and increasing resilience we must first understand that mindfulness is not "a silver bullet for solving all problems facing American Police" (Suttie, 2016). Although not the perfect pill per se, mindfulness can be a beneficial tool for each of us. With the goal of "training our brain to gravitate towards healthy responses, especially in moments of chaos and stress". The treatment has been the subject of hundreds of studies over the past several years, Mindfulness based stress reduction has proved beneficial in reducing stress, anxiety, pain, and depression.

The crux of the mindfulness debate or therapy includes an easy series of meditation practices which promote officer wellness (BJA, 2023). With the intended outcome being resilience and level-headedness, the art of breathing and concentration renders the end user with a broadened ability to think clearly and reduce stress. Not unlike the defensive tactic concept of tactical breathing, if we foster the power of the mind, our body will follow, and our survivability will be enhanced.

I had preached the tactical breathing theory over and over again with each new class I taught. Although grasping the concept fully, I had seldom needed to use it in the field. That all changed one summer night in Missouri. My chief of police and I had been called to a local bar where a large group of tourists and local had been engaged in a fight. Upon our arrival the fight had for the most part subsided with the exception of one large local man. Within a short time, it was determined that no amount of de-escalation absent arrest was going to calm the male or the situation.

Like clockwork, the chief and I caught glimpse of each other's eyes, and the decision was made to place the intoxicated male into custody. As I reached to place the male into custody "the fight was on". I struggled to maintain my grip on the male because of his size. While repeatedly directing the man to stop resisting, it was apparent that my words were falling on deaf ears as he continued to struggle. The male and I fought for a time as the Chief's attention was taken up by the man's wife who decided she would fight with him.

Within a short time, I remember "tasting my heartbeat" which because of my experience meant my heart rate had risen to an unsustainable rate. If I didn't act quickly, the rest of my body would soon activate defensive measures intended to preserve itself, rendering me unable to continue the present fight, likely opening myself up for injury or even worse. Instantly, my mind raced to the training I had taught days before. My words to students of "control your breathing" rang endlessly through my mind. I knew what to do. I had been training others for years. At that moment I began manipulating my body. I began tactically breathing and rapidly slowed my heart rate, allowing me to finish the fight and safely gain the upper hand, ultimately placing the man into custody.

What I had experienced that night was truly nothing more than mindfulness. I recognized a need, felt the negative effects, and countered the negative with positive actions and survived the incident. Likewise, officers who have participated in mindfulness training have reported significantly less anxiety, perceived stress, and post-traumatic stress (BJA, 2023). Later in this chapter we will discuss several mindfulness exercises which officers can benefit from. Understanding that the benefit to the system of mindfulness requires repetition, which can prove challenging. With each class I teach I remind officers that tactical breathing is not something they can just choose to pull out one day and find it successful. Rather, they must practice it to gain the full benefit.

This poses a potential problem for officers because of their busy schedules. Determining when it would be best to practice mindfulness techniques does not have to follow a stringent time from but could easily be implemented into their daily routine. Practicing mindfulness, according to the U.S. Department of Justice can be practiced:

- Before the start of a shift
- After clearing a call
- Before leaving work and arriving home
- During a lunch break or other break at work
- Before going to sleep

The key is repetition and commitment to success.

The concept of mindfulness first became apparent to me during a time I was struggling heavily as the elected Mayor in the small rural town of Winona Missouri, although I had no concept of mindfulness at that point. Rapid changes, infighting and struggling with accomplishing my goals I remember preparing for a city council meeting where I would surely face a major backlash from fellow city officials for doing the right thing. As I patrolled that day, preparing mentally for the evenings meeting, I just couldn't turn my thoughts off.

The thoughts of attending the meeting and having to deal with the discourse wore upon me. It was then that my faith kicked in and I remembered reading a scripture about laying your burdens at the feet of Christ and trusting him to take them. His promise was that He would always be there, walking alongside me and I had no option but to trust that. I don't want to say that I was about to put that promise to the test because that is not what I did. But I was resolved to give it all to Him and trust Him to fix my thoughts. There, in the silence of my patrol car, I began singing. I sang the same old-time hymn, *It Is Well With My Soul,* over and over again for several minutes. Thinking of nothing but the words of the song, I became Intune to what the words were saying and within moments, my angst departed. The meeting came and gone, uneventful, and I learned the true power of not only God but likewise of my mind.

Meditation Exercises (IACP)

Breathing Meditation

Breathing meditation helps the brain learn to observe what is happening in the present.

How to practice it

1. Find a seated position- sit where you are comfortable.

2.   Notice your breath- Bring your attention to how you are breathing. Just breathe naturally. Notice your belly or chest rising.

3.   Slow your breathing- After a few breaths begin to slow down your inhalation and exhales. Focus on making your exhale longer than your inhale. Try counting to make it easier.

4.   Monitor your thoughts- The goal is to focus your attention gently on the breath, but as you breathe, you will notice that your mind will wander. This is normal and will continue throughout the meditation.

5.   Refocus your attention on your breath- When you catch your mind wandering notice it but guide your attention back to your breath. It's ok to notice or even think about your thoughts wandering. Notice it but return to your breathing.

What we have just described is one of many mindfulness exercises designed around centering yourself and becoming more aware of what is going on around you. There are ample resources available for officers hoping to benefit from tools similar to this. A resource I once felt was not quite manly enough ended up being a tool which I often use to maintain my professionalism and bearings as I go about my daily life.

Chapter Summary and Key Takeaways

·   Mindfulness can appear emasculating or even "touchy feely" but in reality, it is simply about focus.

·   Mindfulness relates to reducing stress and increasing resilience.

·   Although not a "magic pill" or "silver bullet", mindfulness can be a beneficial tool for officers hoping to reduce stress.

·   Ridding ourselves of negative thoughts can many times be accomplished through meditation.

Chapter Sixteen

Faith Factor

"Faith is the first factor in a life devoted to service. Without it, nothing is possible. With it, nothing is impossible."

~ Mary McLeod Bethune

A s I sat on the hillside overlooking the ballfields at Columbine High School my mind wandered. Before me lay a mass of humanity. It seemed as though the entire community had come out to try and catch a glimpse of what had occurred less than twenty-four hours before. Behind me, the carnage left by two boys determined to harm others. My job that day was simple. My team and I were tasked with the side security of the school, ensuring that no one entered the property. This aspect, securing the crime scene, was essential to ensure that the investigators on scene had nothing to worry about but the job before them. As I looked out over the pure mass of people I watched as some cried, some stricken with silence and many others simply stood in awe over what had occurred. Behind me, I noticed a cross, erected in remembrance.

Standing my post, I recall the enormity of what had occurred flowing over me. Absent any words sufficient to describe the feeling all I could muster was the thought that I hoped God eased the pains of the families and community. For me, I had little doubt that He was present and walking alongside, even holding this community which suffered so much that day. My belief was placed within me early in life and although I, like most, have stumbled along the way, I have often felt the presence of God in my life, carrying me through my darkest hours.

Not unlike me and my experiences, many men, and women within the law enforcement and first responder communities have relied on what we call the faith factor to carry us through our darkest hours and biggest struggles. Anyone who has laced on the boots or pinned on a badge can attest to the fact that over time we can easily become jaded. As described by Cary Friedman (2016) "officers experience years of exposure to human suffering and evil, an often critical and unappreciative public, corruption, and injustice". All these factors can take a heavy toll on the men and women destined to serve.

Regardless of whether you serve in a large metropolitan department or a small rural community, the experiences and confrontations are the same. I used to believe that policing was different depending upon the officer's demographic region or size of his or her community. As I have grown in experience, I now assert that policing is similar for all genres of locations, with each providing a series of unique indicators of citizenry and workflow. When confronted with a shooter, determined to escape at all costs, whether I'm seeking cover behind a dumpster, or an oak tree bears little significance. Likewise, the demographic data surrounding the neighborhood means nothing while holding the lifeless body, trying to breathe life back into a six-month old child who had been starved to death and horrendously beaten by her mother. What matters at that moment is how we can possibly keep the event in perspective to ensure we live and thrive another day.

For a multitude of men and women serving that meaning or perspective has been found in their faith. For me it is my faith in God, for others it may be their faith in Buddha, Allah, Confucius, their family, their wife, or their job. The faith factor often seen throughout the Law enforcement culture is not determined by one singular point of reason but rather whatever the individual officer deems is worthy of their faith. It is the one concept which allows the individual to rest upon when times get difficult. The key is that the officer finds something or someone to have faith in. The Faith Factor, as I call it is an essential part of resilience and maintaining a positive attitude regardless of the situation faced.

For the officer pinned down, awaiting back up, his or her faith may mean the difference of surviving or not. Likewise, seeing the things we see on a daily basis can cause us to fall into a chasm of hopelessness, questioning why and how evil can exist on such a large level. It is common for officers to become fixated on the tragedy, questioning the purpose of continuing on. The Faith Factor allows the officer to find reasoning behind actions and enhances our ability to move forward in spite of the tragedy, keeping the entirety of the situation in perspective.

Through many recent studies pertaining to faith as it relates to law enforcement type work, "many officers reported feeling comfort in or obtaining a surge of strength from their faith or relationship with God" (Pitel, Marian et.al., 2018). One officer described "I asked God to be with me... God is the reason I didn't get shot. The gunman shot at me several times but missed. I know that it is because God protected me".

A person's faith is an imperative factor for how they carry out their duties each day. Not only does their faith contribute to their interactions with others but also to their willingness to sacrifice for others. Regardless of whether a person has placed their faith in God or themselves, their commitment to their belief system molds their every interaction. For a born again Christian, their faith is founded upon the principle of sacrifice. God sent his son to this world to save the world by being the sacrificial lamb per se. To atone for mankind's sin. The grace, supplied by God through His Son Jesus, allows you and me to accept this gift and be assured of atonement and eternal life. All we have to do is ask. Once we ask and accept, we become new. Never again to risk condemnation because our fate is sealed.

So how does the belief system of Christianity relate to the modern law enforcement officer and the faith factor? Simple, the relation is all encompassing. Does it mean once a person accepts Christ that all of their worries and pain will subside, no. What it means is that upon accepting Christ, you never again walk alone. Our understanding of what is going on around us takes on a new perspective. Where I once felt fear, I now feel that although I may still be afraid, I am not at it alone. I can be confident in my ultimate outcome so the present outcomes bear lesser significance. In a sense, I have less to worry about and more understanding as I strive to remain grounded throughout my duties.

With the assumption that most of our ideas and behaviors stem from our faith our habits are likewise many times grounded in our belief system. A persons strongly held beliefs or faith allows them to become confident in their feelings of truth, values, and the basic good in people. Faith is the means by which many find security and meaning as they confront the darkness surrounding them. Broken down to its simplest form, faith or the lack there in is the foundation for how a person views the world around them.

As we remain determined to provide effective tools for overcoming the trauma and stress so often experienced within each law enforcement officer, I believe our faith factor is an imperative component to success. I do not say this with the singular notion of faith but the all-inclusiveness of the faith factor. As I discussed earlier in this chapter, it is imperative that each person find that one thing that they find faith in. I have met officers who have a strongly held faith in God and officers who have had strong faith in themselves and their abilities. Each seemingly effective approaches to sustained resilience.

I met an officer years ago who for the most part had no recognizable faith in any outside being or deity. Rather, his faith lay within himself. When he was confronted by suffering and pain, he simply retreated within himself and found purpose for what he was seeing. As he experienced great joy from witnessing kind actions, he humbled himself and inspired him to mirror the actions. His stringent yet uplifting childhood had conditioned him not only to recognize the bad things around him but also to center wholly on the greater good of community, fair play, and purposeful living. His resounding faith in his abilities and experience assisted him with overcoming several rather hairy situations, coming out unscathed along the way.

Similarly, I know a man who whole heartedly places his faith in God and God alone. Although far from the textbook, stereotypical, often described "good Christian Boy", my friend stumbled quite readily. He cussed on occasion, looked lustfully at some women, and even was known to cheat on card games every now and then while he drank a beer with his friends. Far from perfect, my friend is, yet totally forgiven and a work in progress according to him. His foundation is his belief that although flawed, he has a constant companion he can turn to and find guidance through.

When confronted with angry words, my friend fights back his desire to return the words in kind. He told me once that the only way he has been able to find solace was through his knowledge that God's plan was perfect. His faith not only sets the tone by which my friend is able to make it through difficult times, but it also helps him choose what is the best path to take when striving to curb behavior, meet the needs of others, and resolve problems. Without faith, my friend would be lost, in his words, it is the anchor by which he keeps from drifting.

A third friend approaches the faith factor in a similar yet much different way. Although strongly raised in his faith the officer rests upon the promises God has made to him as well as all others who choose to welcome Him into their lives. As a young child of eleven, my friend was invited to stay over at the home of his family's minister's home. He was excited to have the opportunity to hang out with the minister's teenage son because to be quite honest, the guy was pretty cool.

As the evening turned into darkness, the illusions of grandeur were realized and the boy had a great time, learning about all the cool things teenagers did. As the evening came to a close and the children headed off to bed the night took a totally different turn. That night my friend was sexually assaulted under the guise of friendship and experimentation. Looking back, he described that it was evident that what occurred had was nothing new for this older boy and my friend wondered how many other victims were out there. Feeling embarrassed and yet unsure if what had occurred was legally wrong, although in his mind, unnatural, the young boy still had the desire of not wanting to get the older boy in trouble.

My friend became resolved to simply put what happened behind him and he really never thought about it until he entered the field of law enforcement. What could have easily become the means by which this young man could deny that God existed and if He did, definitely didn't look out for His children, my friend did the opposite. Maturing in his faith, my friend was able to keep the incident in perspective. Although inappropriate and wrong, God hadn't committed the offense. Rather, God carried him through, paving the path for what one young man would become. To this day, my friend remains focused on God and His teachings.

Which is right? Who is wrong? Or possibly, is there a truth which lies within all these stories? In the end, the important factor is not who a person's faith rests upon but that it rests upon something or someone. When a person finds faith in something their ability to overcome is broadened. With faith, our ability to cope with the day-to-day stressors of the calling are heightened. The Faith Factor provides a foundation by which effective resolution can be made.

Chapter Summary and Key Takeaways

· Many law enforcement officers rely on a faith factor as a means not only to cope with difficult situations but also as a guide for their daily interactions and decision making.

· Where a person's faith factor rests is unimportant. The importance rests in the fact that a person has faith in something or someone.

· The faith factor is an effective tool for overcoming tragedy and coping with everyday stressors.

· A person's faith molds the person's beliefs and behaviors.

Chapter Seventeen

Risk of Non-Healthy Methods of Coping

"if you dare nothing, then when the day is over, nothing is all you will have
gained"

~Neil Gaiman

Many times, in law enforcement we are conditioned to take calculated risks. Whether it's directing traffic, at night, along a ice covered roadway, plunging into a iced over river to save a life, or entering a doorway not knowing who was waiting on the other side, risks are a part of our calling. They always have been and always will be. Regardless of the conditions, timing, or our feelings, we assume the risks of service and move forward in hopes of solving society's problems while maintaining peace and order.

Modern officers are not unlike the leather clad sheriffs of old, entering into the dust-filled saloon not knowing who or what they would face. Be it the first law enforcement officers or the modern-day warrior, the profession carries with it extreme risk. Outside the common risks of injury or death by the hands of an intruder, automobile accidents, and work-related exposure, officers face a much more dangerous foe. The foe of complacency where our own physical and mental health is concerned can, like other risks, prove catastrophic.

I walked into the Sheriff's Office and immediately walked into my personal office and shut the door. Being a people pleaser was just not in the cards today. The overwhelming sense of tiredness and disappointment overtook every portion of my mind. After twenty-nine years of doing my best to serve the communities I had served in, what was I left with? What had I accomplished? Nothing, I thought. It was all in vain. I gave my blood sweat and tears to my brothers and sisters and this profession only to experience my payback. A payback of discontent and lies. As I reached to remove the proverbial knife from my back, I had lost count of the knives I had removed previously, long before. I was tired with no relief in sight.

As I sat at my desk my mind wandered to everything I had done for this place, for this community, for these people. Why would I be repaid in this fashion? Weren't my brothers and sisters supposed to have my back? Wasn't good supposed to prevail? Why couldn't I pull myself out of this? I'm so tired!

I remember that day like it was yesterday. I had reached an all-time low in life. Sure, I had faced troubling times before, times where it was difficult to keep my mind straight. This time seemed different. This time I couldn't escape the confines of my mind. Over twenty-nine years of service, coupled with years of ineffectively coping with the trauma and stress I had encountered had finally surfaced. I could no longer simply push the trauma to the back burner of my mind because to be quite frank, it was full. What happened next, although difficult, was minor considering how some officers are forced to deal with the demons they have held inside for so long.

For me, the risks of not adequately addressing my own mental health simply caused me to end my career. For many others, the result is far more severe, including a loss of relationships, faith and even life. As one brother-in-law enforcement described "My wife and I started fighting over the dumbest stuff. I would get so mad over little things, and it was affecting our perfect life". Another brother describes "During my career, I'm not proud of it but I had affairs. It's not that I searched for a tryst outside my marriage, and sex was never the goal, I couldn't find solace in my marriage and sought out friends who understood me and my job. The affairs turned to feelings of guilt, causing me to hate myself even more".

One of the unfortunate results or risks of unchecked trauma in our lives is the fact that our relationships can suffer. Studies depict that fifty-three percent of law enforcement marriages end in divorce. Is this number a result of trauma? The answer is unknown but a viable option in my opinion. As our fellow officers have described it's difficult to turn it off sometimes. I remember my second wife describing, in a fit of anger, that she would never date a cop again. My reply was simple, uncaring, and precise... why because you don't want to get caught again? I asked. What made this response so unique is that I never spout off responses. I have become known for my calmness and collectedness regardless of any situation. Similarly, for me to respond so uncaringly to the woman I truly loved was concerning.

Although I've never felt that my career or the stress therein caused marital turmoil for me in my marriage, I can recognize that certain aspects of my relationships had been affected. I had become hardened to a certain point; it flowed over at times. I remember speaking to my second wife shortly after we decided to separate. She voiced her frustration over my willingness to call it quits with no attempt to rescue the marriage. In my mind, I wasn't going to beg, I wasn't going to chase. I would sit silently, struggling internally to cope with the loss I felt would end me. I had become a master at hiding emotion and unbeknownst to me it showed in my marriage. Her response was rapid and remains vivid to me, "You fought for fourteen years for your first marriage but not at all for us". She was right, although I was struggling inside, I refused to let it show. Not unlike my first wife saying "you never show emotion, I've never seen you cry" I simply carried on.

The risk of fractured and lost relationships is one of many potential hazards of failing to effectively cope with trauma and stress. So often officers risk falling into the chasm they cannot climb out of because of the stress in their lives. Attempting to soften the pain they experience through unhealthy habits such as unhealthy eating, drugs, and alcohol abuse can many times temporarily fill the void caused by ineffective coping. One officer describes "I spent six months drinking heavily; it helped by not allowing me to sleep so I could avoid the nightmares I experienced."

Another brother described that he struggled with dealing with a major critical incident and his recovery. He shared that life became somewhat a blur to him where all he truly wanted to do was sit on the couch and watch the television. His wife and kids became distant to him because he truly hadn't come to grips with how to deal with the pent-up trauma he had experienced throughout his career.

Entering the career of law enforcement, we somewhat understand the risks we will be facing. We fully understand that we may be called upon to run towards gunfire, into a burning building, or step between two feuding parties. The inward struggle when confronted with risks for the most part is absent. Every officer knows the risks and accepts that although they love life and seldom want to risk not going home at night, our calling may one day require it, to ensure that others may live. What we fail to truly understand is that the risk of unresolved trauma is many times greater than the risk of a bad guy with a gun or a drunk behind the wheel.

Chapter Summary and Key Takeaways

· Risks are an ever-present and common factor within the law enforcement community and career as well as many other first responder professions.

· Professionals who fail to adequately confront their unresolved trauma and stress will many times experience fractures in their lives both professionally and personally.

· Failing to implement effective coping strategies can many times leave officers with failing marriages, fractured relationships, and a wide array of other negative aspects associated with a build up of stress and unresolved trauma.

· Poor coping mechanisms including drug or alcohol abuse, poor nutrition, solitude, and a negative outlook are many times the result.

· Many fail to recognize the enormity of the risk we face with unresolved trauma and stress.

Chapter Eighteen

Organizations With the Mission to Help

"If you're out there and need help, seek it. Be proud of your valiant day-to-day struggle. There is no shame in needing support."

~Jared Padalecki

I sat, wondering if my fellow brothers and sisters knew about the help that was out there? Help designed to broaden their perspective about not only work-related stressors but likewise about the daily struggles of life outside the workplace. For so many years, throughout my career, I knew nothing about behavioral health support. Sure, we routinely encountered citizens who struggled, and had the process down for getting them help, pretty well. My knowledge of the system really stopped there. Would I ever treat a fellow brother or sister or even myself to the help I recognized? Absolutely not.

My reluctance wasn't because we or I were any better than the citizens we served or that the "help" was subpar, it was because I fully understood the ramifications of such actions. For an officer to check themselves into a hospital or be subjected to a mental health hold, it would be career ending. All of their hard work, aspirations, and future desires would immediately come to a screeching halt with one simple stroke of the pen. Hence, in my mind there was no need nor any viable benefits to seeking help, even if I needed it. Myself and my brothers and sisters would simply carry on as we always had and surely overcome in the end.

It was only through the persistence of my local behavioral health professionals and my own commitment to research that I learned I was wrong and that there is a wide variety of not only help available to officers but likewise benefits therein. As my region's community behavioral health liaison persisted with his commitment of bringing help to law enforcement officials, I rapidly began to reach a heightened level of understanding. Not only was there help for those unfortunate citizens who struggle with stress and mental health conditions, there also has become a movement to serve those who serve their communities daily.

Over the last several years the concept of first responder mental health and wellbeing has come to the forefront of discussion, causing a great emphasis to be placed on first responder mental health and ending the stigma's associated with reaching out for help and support.

As I spoke to a classroom full of law enforcement officers it was apparent that we were beginning to see a positive shift in understanding. Where we once felt reluctant to even confront the issue of mental health, we now for the most part accept it and seek out ways to address not only the solutions but likewise the underlying causes. How did we get here? Simple, through hard work and persistence on the part of numerous individuals, groups, organizations, and associations. Although definitely not all inclusive, I would like to take a few moments and discuss several of the modern-day concepts we have been utilizing to bring the issue of mental wellness to the forefront of our minds and to provide assistance to officers in their time of need.

As I have described, for me, my knowledge was enhanced through the work of one man primarily. This man happened to be simply doing his job. In the state of Missouri, the Department of Mental Health, through changes in the procedures surrounding mental health enacted an innovative program. The program would entail designating regional Community Behavioral Health Liaisons, first known as Community Mental Health Liaisons, who would be tasked with not only working with citizens who were experiencing mental health crisis's but also working alongside local law enforcement officer. Their duty would be to help officers understand behavioral health more effectively which in turn would equip the officers with a broader knowledge and capabilities to effectively deal with citizens experiencing crisis.

Additionally, the Community Behavioral Health Liaison would be tasked with educating those same law enforcement officers in areas surrounding their own mental health, coping strategies, and the importance of wellness. One of the primary education goals for the community behavioral health liaison was to train and implement the concept of Crisis Intervention Teams throughout the State of Missouri. With the goals of training officers in how to recognize potential indicators that a person is suffering from mental illness and or going through a mental health or substance use crisis, the officer is better equipped to effectively deal with the situation.

In addition to training officers in recognizing possible indicators of mental illness, broadening their perspective in de-escalations tactics as they relate to mental illness related crisis and how to potentially communicate and address the crisis is a major emphasis. These factors coupled with Crisis Intervention Teams inherent desire to enhance the officer's own wellness and resilience while simultaneously adding to their tools for use in the field, makes for a win -win for officer safety both internally and externally.

Another beneficial concept / organization which has made great strides in enhancing officer wellness is the inclusion of programs such as the Critical Incident Management Seminars and Post Critical Incident Management Seminars. I had become aware of critical incident management while serving as the Sheriff in Carter County Missouri. Early in my term chatter had begun through the industry about the benefits to holding post incident debriefings. An open time of discussion and planning officers were able to discuss incidents and explore what went right and what went wrong. The benefits were huge in my opinion although the concept was not new to me.

Early in my career, I had a co-worker and supervisor who encouraged me, as well as others, to take a moment after each call and think about what had occurred. When it was safe, he would say, think about how it all went... what was good, what was bad.... What was safe and not so safe. Then, he would say, think about how we can do it better, safer. Grasping what he was saying, the concept became a ritual for me and for years, when I was safe, I would run each event through my mind and do just as he said.

Following the same guides for the most part, the benefits of debriefing are countless. Understanding the benefits to not only evaluating what occurred and telling our story, the concept of Post Critical Incident Management Seminars has exploded in many states, paving the way to true healing. The Missouri State Highway Patrol recognized a need to provide a forum by which officers and their families could not only confront trauma but also learn strategies to overcome. The Success of PCIMS type seminars have become so overwhelming many organizations and agencies are beginning to design their own programs with similar results in mind.

Likewise, organizations such as the Missouri Crisis Intervention Team Council and Department of Mental Health have recognized the need for resources which will make seeking assistance not only easier for officers serving their communities but also more palatable for officers to take that leap and utilize the services.

One such vision turned reality is Missouri's First Responder Network. Understanding that finding the perfect fit as therapy or counselors are concerned is difficult for many first responders, the networks' goal is to provide information relating to vetted professionals centered on the first responder community. Coming to the realization that first responders benefit highly from receiving services from a man or woman who understands their calling, the first responder network is made up of only clinicians who show not only competence in the field but likewise a desire to work alongside law enforcement and first responder professionals to accomplish joint goals.

The first responder network is a service where each practitioner undergoes an exhaustive vetting process to ensure that they are equipped and qualified to be listed in the database. First responders can locate the network through simply conducting a world wide web search or responds to www.missouricit.org/first-responders. Once on the site, officers and first responders can see a listing of clinicians throughout the state of Missouri who specialize in assisting first responders.

Another useful tool taking the first responder community by storm is the use of cellular telephone apps designed to immediately provide helpful resources to first responders and law enforcement officers on demand. One such application was rolled out in the State of Missouri, in 2022. The Cordico Wellness app is a tool where officers can download a cell phone-based application which they can utilize to retrieve not only the latest research and data about a wide array of mental health disorders they likewise can benefit from tips and tools for healthy living, nutrition, fitness, mental toughness, and numerous self-assessments. The app touts a wellness toolkit with over sixty topics covering not only articles, but videos designed for ease of distribution.

As with the State of Missouri, many states across our country and world have made it a priority to begin centering upon the wellness and resiliency of the first responder and law enforcement communities. One of the easiest manners by which an officer can locate the resources available throughout your own state is to contact your states Department of Mental Health for directions or the States Crisis Intervention Team Council.

In addition to the resources which have been made available within your state, numerous organizations have developed programs designed to aid when officers are in a time of need. Below is a brief list of some resource points available to first responders and Law Enforcement officers.

Law Enforcement Survival Institute

P.O. Box 297

Westminster, CO. 80036

1-303-940-0411

National Police Suicide Foundation

7015 Clark Road

Seaford, Delaware 19973

1-302-536-1214

1-866-276-4615

SAFE Call Now

P.O. Box 2654

Kirkland, Wa.

1-206-459-3020

Law Enforcement Family Support Network

P.O. Box 32831

Fidley, Mn. 55432

Lawenforcmentfamilysupport.org

Blue Wall Institute

37 Charvel Drive

Belleville, Il 62226

1-618-791-9146

COP Line

1-800-COPLINE

1-800-267-5463

Cop 2 Cop

1-866-Cop-2COP

1800-267-2267

Blue Help

www.bluehelp.org

International Conference of Police Chaplain's

1-850-654-9736

National Police Wives Association

www.admin@nationalpolicewivesassociation.org

First Responder Treatment

1-888-979-2176

CopsAlive.com

Chapter Summary and Key Takeaways

·   Stressors stem from a wide variety of sources outside the workplace as well as inside. Stressors including family or relationship strife, financial issues, and social stigma can add to an officer's overall outlook and stress level.

·   A reluctance to seek help remains within many throughout the first responder and law enforcement community. Although a great deal of work has been done to lower the stigmas surrounding mental health, we must remain vigilant if we hope to affect a true change of mindset.

·   There are numerous organizations developed to assist our law enforcement and first responders. For a person seeking help or simply wishing to provide resources as a good starting point or through contacting your individual states department of mental health or crisis intervention team council.

Chapter Nineteen

Words from the Pack

"The most valuable gift you can receive is an honest friend."
~ Stephan Richards

As the journey to complete the follow-up on my original book, *The Calling* unfolded, a voice of reason came to me from one of my most valued advisors. While discussing my book, my wife turned and began talking with me about the fact that although the genre of my book was not what she typically enjoyed she found it quite interesting. She began describing that although she did not know the severity of everything, I went through she could see the effects my career had on my daily behavior. As we spoke, this kind and ultra intelligent woman interjected saying "the only problem is you exposed the need but really didn't do enough with discussing the remedy".

As we talked, I thought about the countless hours which went into preparing and developing the concepts behind the book coupled with our goals of not only providing the readers with a glimpse into the mind of law enforcement officers and the battles they face. My wife's vision was directly in line with mine and the second book was conceived. My wife went on to make one request. She explained "don't be clinical, be real". This perfect woman in five short words had captured the true meaning of what it would take to reach our desired audience. As we know, cops are very intelligent but prefer a sort of realness when we speak. And if we hoped to affect true change and provide a tool which could be useful, we would need to be real.

My wife elaborated on her statement and requested that in the second book, we interview and add to our content the words from real officers. Officers who struggle, fight, and overcome daily throughout our communities. With this concept in mind, I thought that there was truly no better way to wrap this book up than through the words of advice from your brothers and sisters in blue.

As we strive to honor our calling both at work and on the home front, wisdom stems from the hearts and minds of those who have walked along the same path. When asked to provide our readers with tips for surviving the career of law enforcement, A dear friend and long-time brother in the field describes:

We must find a life outside law enforcement. It is a must. Find a hobby. If you are married, find a way to fall in love with your bride every day. Please don't sacrifice your wife or husband and your kids at the alter of law enforcement.

Take time off, giving yourself permission to take a mental health day every now and then. Many times, especially in small departments, guilt gets in the way because you don't want to let your partners down. Listen, there is no special rewards for being Mr. or Mrs. Iron man or woman or having that year where we did not take a single day off. Screw that! We are talking about your health here, and your family's health. I worked on a domestic violence once that took me into the next day of my vacation that I had planned with my family. I was worthless because I was up for over twenty-four hours, so my family suffered and I could never calm down, relax, or decompress. My trip began with me being angry. I was running late and that was huge for me. Looking back, I could've asked a colleague to help, and they would have... but I was too proud.

Having a more work- life balance, again, might mean taking time off. No sense in banking your accrued time to max, I lost four hundred plus hours of six time leave when I retired.

Above all, Get Help! When we are sick with bronchitis, strep, etc. we go to the doctor and get antibiotics. Why shouldn't we do the same when our mind and mental health are sick? This isn't a bad thing. There is nothing wrong with you. Your mind can only take so much BS from the dregs of human nature. I don't think we are wired to clean up suicide after suicide. We are not wired to fight off some drug induced jerk-off that has grabbed our holster and is trying to yank your service weapon out, all the while looking at this individual and you swear, you're looking at Satan himself.

We are not wired to hold young people on an accident scene as they take agonal breaths after their bodies have been ripped open like a stuffed toy and you hold them as they pass on to eternity. Our minds become unwell after seeing one, or unfortunately, a whole career of all those things combined. You must get to a doctor ASAP to help you unravel our mind and get our heads working straight again.

For my retired brothers and sisters don't retire. Ok, retired from law enforcement but not from life and not from being productive. We are created to move and produce. We must have a game plan. Expect to have an identity crisis. This doesn't mean you have to have a crisis but there will be self-questioning. Also don't hesitate to get counseling, just because you're not in it doesn't mean you're still not dealing with it.

Another sister describes:

If you are mentally burnt out because of your job, do not stay in it until it breaks you. This job is not worth your life. Either find a new career or change of pace within the law enforcement field. I eventually realized that if I stayed in law enforcement my mental health was going to suffer. I began to investigate other careers and other areas within law enforcement where I could make more of a difference. The change to a different position within law enforcement that I chose isn't for everyone but for me it was my saving grace.

When you are off duty, be just that. Do not take this job home with you, rather find a way to communicate with your family, especially on the hard days. Take care of your childhood trauma before the weight of this job starts eating away at your mental health. Eventually, you will work a case that snaps you right back into that trauma. And of course, do not isolate yourself from loved ones and stay physically active. My mental health always takes a spiral downwards if I slack on my physical health. I must be very vigilant on staying up with my physical health and remaining social with family and friends or my mental health begins to decay.

Another fellow Law Enforcement brother describes "I would recommend anyone dealing with any incident which is wearing on them, to get help. I couldn't deal with it myself. I've heard it takes a real man to ask for help and I truly believe there is some truth to that statement".

One long term retiree from law enforcement began telling me about his life and wanted to impart his belief and thoughts upon all those within the field of service. He describes:

Listen, life sucks sometimes. We don't go into this job hoping for pain, sorrow, and nightmares. Unfortunately, that is exactly what we get right alongside the happiness, joy, and pride in saving lives and affecting change. Be the change and be willing to open your eyes to the possibility of getting help. Not unlike the tactical planning you learned to fine tune over the years. We have to be able to think outside the box and adjust when necessary.

I remember sitting outside a house during a routine warrant service call, when a voice was heard our tactics had to change and we sprang into action. Just like that, when the voice deep inside us is telling us that something is wrong, we must adjust what we are doing in order to successfully complete the mission. There is no disgrace in retreating to gain a better tactical position and there is no disgrace in seeking to silence those voices.

Take the time to get in tune with yourself. Find your foundation and seek to always rest upon it. Be there for your family and give them the same fervor you give your job. I lost my first marriage because my job was everything to me. Being a cop was all I ever wanted, and it ended up being all I was left with. My children despised me, and I had no friends because I was always the skeptic in the room. I had to learn that life must be placed on a pedestal and those we care about and love, must be emphasized as important. It wasn't until I sought help and got back to my faith that I truly experienced peace, the kind of peace I had been trying to bring to the communities I served for decades.

If I could give every cop one word of advice it would simply be that although the cop life is not about them, about how cool they look, or as big and bad they are, or the power and control they exert, their health is. What we officers must understand is that our calling is about the service to our community and fellow man and our mission is only accomplished through awareness. Awareness not only in the constant desire to remain updated on tactics and law but also in our own resilience. A resilience which is foundationally based upon our ability and willingness to recognize and counter any foe we may encounter. Even if that foe happens to be our own mind.

Chapter Twenty

Commitment to the Mission

"Outstanding people have one thing in common: an absolute sense of mission."

~Zig Ziglar

In Dr. Kevin M. Gilmartin's Ph.D. book Emotional Survival for Law Enforcement (2002) he provides vivid descriptions of how many officers begin their career with enthusiasm, energy, and commitment. Careers which end after years of serving with the same officer becoming cynical, divorced, and alienated from family and friends. In the same book Dr. Gilmartin described officers who experienced a different outcome. Outcomes where the officer retained their core values and whose relationships thrived. The difference between the two rests solely upon those officers and the steps they took to counter the negative aspects of the field. Steps through which they developed strategies to keep healthy, strengthen their mind and body, bolster their relationships and increase focus on their own spiritual health.

Time after time, resource after resource, one can find evidence of the benefits of establishing a proactive resolution process for dealing with the day-to-day traumas associated with law enforcement and first responder type work. Failure to fully understand the impact of unresolved trauma and not addressing it appropriately will surely leave us with few options other than struggling to remain afloat in a world of constantly rising water. Addressing our own mental health is similar in my mind to many of the incidents, situations, and calls we face. All of which are proved more difficult absent a clear mission.

When I became more and more confident in my ability to serve my community as a police officer the concept of mission planning began to surface. Sure, I had read all the departmental or organizational "mission statements" along the way and even signed my name along the signature line attesting to my compliance many times. Could I recite them today? Could I share them with another? Not hardly. They were simply no more than words on paper. Words designed to check some procedural box that administrators could hold against us. Although understandably important, they simply held little importance to me.

I had lost sight of those old war movies I found inspiration in as a child. Those same movies which depicted the worn team of men who although tired, hurt, worn and weathered, maintained the mission at hand. Through sickness and health, rain or shine, they moved across enemy terrain avoiding gun fire and mortars all in hope of meeting their goal and finishing their mission. Not unlike those old movies we too have a mission. A mission filled with moments where we may encounter difficult terrain, enemy fire, and hazards littering the roadway. A mission by which we must maintain focus and fulfill our destiny.

A mission is described as "an important goal or purpose that is accompanied by strong conviction, a calling". One Sheriff's Office lists their mission statement as follows: "We take pride in providing professional law enforcement service by enhancing the quality of life through community interaction and partnerships, prevention of crime and efficient service to the public". For anyone inside the calling of service known as law enforcement it is a given that our purpose or mission per se is to provide professional services designed around preventing crime and enhancing opportunities.

What must occur is that each of us ensure that it is our personal purpose or mission to carry that mission over to not only our communities and the public but likewise to our brothers and sisters in law enforcement and even ourselves. Where enhancing the quality of life of our citizens is important, similarly, enhancing our own quality of life bears huge significance. Prevention of crime is imperative while prevention of loss through suicide and stress related non-retention of our brothers and sisters is likewise significant. Being committed to the mission of resiliency must become a widely known and staple of our everyday lives.

So how do we become committed as a group to change the police culture to reflect a commitment to the mission of enhancing officer wellness and resiliency? It all begins with our desire to take a stand and become "real", understanding that although the topic is void many times of comfort, it is necessary and essential. This commitment begins with each of us. Every officer, deputy, dispatcher, fire fighter, first responder, emergency medical worker, and supervisor must make it their mission to put aside the proverbial stigmas associated with mental health and make it our mission to change.

Our mission must include making mental health and effective coping mechanisms a part of our everyday lives. Make it routine even. Creating an atmosphere where seeking help or voicing concern is welcomed with support and resources rather than cringes. This transition is not an easy one. As I described earlier in this offering, it's easy to welcome or recommend resilience and even resources available to everyone else. It's much more difficult to recognize the need deep within ourselves.

Our mission or commitment to changing the police culture relating to our own mental health must carry with it a desire to become self-aware and assertive. How? As we discussed through a shift in mindset. When I became aware of everything out there for my people, I shifted from an attitude of reaction to that of action. To fully thrive I needed to make that action inclusive of myself. To do that I simply had to do what I did every day, I had to begin making me a priority, making my safety a priority just like I did for my co-workers and citizens. I had to begin understanding that although I was strong, it was more than acceptable to seek help. It was ok to reach out for the many safety lines that floated in the waters around me.

Chapter Twenty-One

Conclusion

"it's ok daddy, you can cry."
~Riyann Stephens

M y family has grown over the years. Not only in number and size but also in those areas seldom seen in public. We have prided ourselves in building not only strength, faith, and resilience within ourselves. But a strong family unit who can lean on each other when the times get difficult. Recently this strength has become more than apparent through the words of my nine- year-old daughter. To truly benefit from the story, one must go back several years to a much younger, much fitter me.

As a young child my parents, and honestly, more so me, benefited from a friendship with a Colorado State Trooper. My dad became friends with Stan years before while he, dad, was an over the road truck driver. At some point my parents had the opportunity to adopt a retired Colorado State Highway Patrol K-9. When Barron became a member of the family, I was not only astonished by his golden coat but the beauty and demeanor of this aging golden German Shepard dog.

Within seemingly moments Baron and I experienced a strong bond based upon friendship. He would run alongside me, wrestle, and even become a soft pillow to rest my weary head upon all while lending a listening ear to a boy struggling to find himself in this life. The times this mountain of a dog ensured the safety of my family, and our friends were too numerous to count. I grew to learn there was no better protector and when I became a parent myself the only true security option was the German Shepherd. Although Baron was my first, he was not the last in the breed owned by me. I simply loved them and considered all other breeds lessor.

When I met my wife, she had quite the opposite thought on pets. Although a sincere pet lover like me, she went the other route and preferred smaller breeds. The toy poodle was her pet of choice. Understanding that no true, strong, warrior type man, let alone a six-foot-seven, two-hundred- fifty pound one, would be caught dead holding a poodle, let alone a toy poodle, I simply grinned and pled my case for the warrior class breed.

Isie was my wife's little baby. A two-pound toy poodle with a permanent grin affixed to her face, left no question of her status within the family unit. She was truly a momma's girl and although she kind of liked me, she made it painfully clear that momma was her human. Although always inclusive, it was obvious that absent my awesome body massages she could do without me as long as she had her momma. Over the years Isie grew on me and the two of us built a bond. My wife brought home a second poodle and it was obvious who wore the pants in our family from that day forth.

Our new poodle, Brie, was smaller in stature than Isie yet had the disposition of the German Shepards I grew to love. Deciding that I would be the lucky one to be her human, Brie and I grew closer and closer with each passing day. My love for the breed grew and although my love for Shepards remains I now have a similarly strong love for the toy poodle.

As our family has grown with time the unfortunate reality of age creeps in. This past year, as I spoke earlier, this aspect became more than real for us. At fourteen, the strong, healthy Isie began experiencing heart issues. Within a span of two weeks, no amount of medication or veterinarian visits seemed to help. This once vibrant girl was lowered to constantly experiencing heart attacks each time, she exited her bed. Not being able to say goodbye to our beloved family member, each time she fell away, I would swoop her up and revive her, compressing her chest and breathing life back into her snout, hoping only that the medication would begin working, providing comfort to Isie and our family.

After two weeks, as difficult as it was, my wife and I made the decision that our constant reviving of Isie was truly not fair to the little girl. Having her with us for one more day was causing her pain and although it hurt greatly, we didn't want her to have to go through that. My wife and I decided that the next time she passed out we would simply let nature take its course and begin the process of grieving our loss. It was determined that when she fell, I would swoop her up and retreat to another room so I could provide any comfort possible and not allow our girls to witness Issues death.

The next evening, Isie entered into another episode. As planned, I picked her up and moved quickly into an adjacent room where I gently stroked her auburn hair and thanked her for the love, she had shown us over the years. Like clockwork Issie stopped breathing and I just held her. After approximately one minute she again began breathing on her own and once she regained her balance, I returned to the living room where I placed her in her mothers' arms. I watched as my girls gathered around their mother doing their best to comfort their mother while restraining their excitement that Isie was still with us.

I did what I have become accustomed to in life, I stepped back, retreated to the comfort of my couch, sat, and just watched. After a short time, my youngest daughter, Riyann walked over to the couch I was seated on. Placing her hand on my shoulder, Riyann looked somberly into my eyes and said, "it's ok daddy" she then said, "it's ok to cry if you want to". Looking at my compassionate child I replied that I was doing alright and thank you. Not accepting my reply, Riyann began patting my shoulder, ever so softly. She then spoke again, "no, it's ok daddy, you're not a cop anymore... its ok to cry and show emotion now".

It has been said that from the mouths of babies we can experience pure truth. On this day that proved true. As I think about little Isie and the purely loving words my child expressed to me, I wonder why so much hesitation is felt on our part to simply be ourselves. Is it the fact that we are raised and grow to be men, be strong, be the ultimate protector? Or is it simply because we are just plain stubborn, and refuse to lower our shields out of fear of exposing the true warrior inside? Either way the last thing we need is for a nine-year-old to recognize a need for emotional wellness before we do.

A major part of becoming and sustaining the strength needed to be a leader in the field of law enforcement is for each of us to follow the example of that little girl and simply let it out. It's a difficult task, but essential.

Chapter Twenty-Two

Appendix

National Resources for Law Enforcement Resiliency

1) Law Enforcement Survival Institute
P.O. Box 297
Westminster, CO 80036
Phone: 1-303-940-0411 Email: lawenforcementsurvivalinstitute.org
Trains law enforcement officers to cope with stress and manage all the toxic effects and hidden dangers of a career in law enforcement.

2) National Police Suicide Foundation
7015 Clark Road
Seaford, Delaware 19973
Phone: 1-302-536-1214; toll free: 1-866-276-4615 Email: redoug2001@aol.com
Confidential suicide hotline for police officers.

3) Safe Call Now
P.O. Box 2654
Kirkland, WA 98083
Phone: 1-206-459-3020 Email: safecallnow.org
Confidential resources and hotline for mental health help for law enforcement and their families.

4) Law Enforcement Family Support Network
P.O. Box 32831
Fridley, MN 55432
Email: myra@lawenforcementfamilysupport.org
Education and support to improve overall health and wellness of law enforcement and their families.

5) First Responder Treatment
Phone: 1-888-979-2176 Email: 1strespondertreatment.com
Counseling and addiction treatment for first responders.

6) Blue Wall Institute
37 Charvel Drive
Belleville, IL 62226
Phone: 1-618-791-9146 Email: bw-institute.com
Provider of first responder holistic wellness training in the areas of health, stress management, suicide prevention, and resiliency training.

LAW ENFORCEMENT STRESS SURVIVAL STRATEGIES
<u>ON DUTY</u>

POWER UP – PREPARE FOR THE MISSION

<u>MENTALLY GEAR UP:</u>
- Just as important as putting on your uniform and protective gear, ready your mind and body for the shift.
- Think about plans, training, procedures/protocols on your way to the duty assignment.
- Take a few moments to mentally rehearse potential scenarios, experiences and challenges that may occur. Also think about your options for reactions, responses and resources.

<u>PLAN AHEAD:</u>
- Fully charge phones and radios.
- Consider taking your own favorite healthy food, snacks, meal, etc.
- Bring additional clothing or supplies if there is an anticipated need (weather issues, etc.).
- Inform your family of anticipated schedule and duties; pre-arrange resources to assist with routine family duties (day care, transportation, meals, etc.) Communicate with family to identify needs and potential people/resources to assist during the time you are on duty.
- Consider talking with family and friends to request minimization of phone calls/texts/emails during duty time. Identify a primary (or several primary) persons/contact(s) with whom you will check-in regularly.

PERFORM – MANAGING THE SHIFT

During a significant event, officers in ALL locations and on ALL assignments confront stress.

<u>PRACTICAL CONSIDERATIONS AND INTERVENTIONS:</u>
- Accept assignment – You may prefer to be at the command center, on the front line, or in your home precinct or zone, but all assignments are essential and important.
- Avoid taking things personally – Use mental armor/protection to keep perspective and reassure yourself that you are simply responding to a situation, you are not personally responsible for the situation or attitudes/behaviors of others. You ARE responsible for your own attitude and behavior.
- Breathe – One of the best strategies for controlling stress, anxiety and promoting healthy physical function is deep breathing. Four cycles of deep inhalation, holding breath, slow exhale and relaxation are effective. Learn and practice with a free app: *TZTB – Tactical Breathing Trainer* by Lieutenant Colonel Dave Grossman.
- Breaks – Take time away to hydrate, get nourishment, stretch and walk/exercise, talk with others, and/or reach out to family ... *rest*.
- Choices – Make good ones! Choose foods, fluids and activities to reduce stress. Use caution with stimulants and minimize foods with highly concentrated sugars and/or fats. Select water, fruit/fruit juices, proteins, etc. Avoid or minimize energy drinks. Free and plentiful are not necessarily good choices.
- Monitor your well-being – Confer with medical resources as needed. Abnormal stress signs and symptoms warranting immediate attention: chest pain, severe shortness of breath, signs of shock (rapid light breathing, quick light pulse, shivering, feeling chilled, nauseated, moist or clammy skin, mental confusion, dilated pupils, freezing up, appearing dazed, severe panic).
- Communicate – Talk with peers and available support personnel, chaplains, etc.
- Speak up – Request assistance or relief for yourself or peers.
- Provide care and concern – Observe and look out for one another.

<u>SHIFTING GEARS – DISENGAGING FROM DUTY:</u>
- Disengaging from an active/intense situation may be challenging as by nature we are action oriented. It is important to break from the incident/situation and not stick around or work extra hours or shifts unless requested to do so.
- Utilize time travelling home to actively engage in mental preparation for wherever you are going. Plan your activities for when you arrive and how you will handle questions or communications.

LAW ENFORCEMENT STRESS SURVIVAL STRATEGIES

OFF DUTY

POWER DOWN -- BALANCE BY PROTECTING AND USING TIME OFF DUTY EFFECTIVELY

- Engage in some transition time if necessary. It is often difficult to go from intense/active situations to relaxation or sleep. For some officers, distracting or refocusing activities are beneficial: reading, watching a movie, playing a game, talking, etc.
- Eat and Sleep. Turn off your phone if possible to get some uninterrupted sleep.
- Exercise within 24 to 48 hours if sufficiently rested.
- Refrain from alcohol consumption as it may interfere with sleep and lowers inhibitions.
- Maintain schedule for medications, meals and health activities.
- Realize that the recovery/balance phase may have a rapid turnaround time, as often shift responsibilities will be 12 hours on and 12 hours off. It is important to use time off duty wisely and efficiently.
- Prepare for potential *normal* reactions to stress: anger, irritability, fatigue, detachment, sleep problems, dreams and nightmares, distractibility, anxiety, worry, frequent thoughts about what has and what may happen, strains in work and personal relationships. Problem-solve and develop an action plan.

BE PROACTIVE – STRESS MANAGEMENT AND RESILIENCE

- Dealing with stress and demands requires ACTION on your part, it doesn't just happen.
- Slow down... take care of yourself.
- Remember that this may be a prolonged situation with disruption in normal routines and activities. Pace yourself for the potential long haul of chronic stress.
- Enlist and accept input and support from family, friends and peers.
- Practice healthy habits: eat well, eat regularly, drink water, rest, exercise and engage in enjoyable activities.
- Talk to people and spend time with others (especially your family).
- Back-up fellow officers and emergency responders by providing support, encouragement and open communication. Sometimes connecting with peers just to talk about thoughts/experiences is most helpful.
- Allocate some dedicated, full-attention time (no cell phone checking/texting/gaming, emailing, etc.) to your spouse/significant other/children/family. Even if it is only a short time to do something normal, eat a meal, play a game, watch a special TV show, etc., they will respond well to uninterrupted time with you. They are experiencing stress too.
- Avoid or minimize exposure to news, media, or frequent discussions/speculations/incident quarterbacking while off duty to assist in truly having a break.
- Don't make any big decisions or life-changing decisions regarding career, relationships, moves, etc. during times of increased stress.
- Have realistic expectations and utilize a problem-solving, practical approach to getting through each day.
- Attend critical incident stress discussions, debriefings and support meetings.
- Utilize personal and professional resources: social support, faith/prayer, clergy, counselors, Employee Assistance Programs, Peer Support Services, Critical Incident Stress Management (CISM) Team.

Grief and Loss

Survival Strategies

❖ **Take care of yourself!-** Take care of your physical needs (eat well, rest, be active, try to avoid things that may impact your nervous system such as caffeine, nicotine, alcohol, etc). If you have difficulty sleeping, try resting in a recliner or chair with your feet elevated. Monitor any physical symptoms and seek medical assessment/treatment if needed.

❖ **Numbness and Shock-** Allow for numbness and shock early in your experience. This reaction is normal and allows you time to gradually deal with loss and allows your emotions to catch up with thoughts and realities.

❖ **Breathing Excercises-** Deep breathing in and out is very effective in reducing stress and anxiety.

❖ **Connect and Communicate Your Need for Help-** Speak from both your head and your heart. Utilize a support system of caring family, friends, peers and professionals. Do not hesitate to speak up and ask for help or inform people what may be helpful to you. If your energy level is low, ask someone to assist you in getting what you need by acting as your advocate.

❖ **Expect to feel a multitude of emotions-** It is normal to experience one or more emotions following the death or loss of someone important to you. You may feel sadness, confusion, fear, guilt, anger, or relief (among others). These emotions may change quickly and may follow each other within a short period of time and is an indicator that your mind and body are reacting normally as a means of coping with your loss.

❖ **It takes time-** What you are experiencing is a normal, human response to grief and loss. Reassure yourself that coping and grieving involves effort time. Over time, your body and mind will begin to stabilize and return to pre-loss functioning. Take things one at a time. Be realistic in your expectations of yourself and others. Return to normal routines and schedule when you feel ready to do so.

❖ **Search for meaning and purpose-** Give some thought to those "Why" and "How" questions, realizing that some of the questions do not have answers. This search for answers is a normal part of seeking explanations for difficult or senseless realities, and working through the questions may help to promote healing.

❖ **Stay active-** Stretching, walking and safety-minded exercise assists in burning off chemicals that our bodies produce as a response to stress. Movement and exercise also promote deep breathing, distraction from your pain, and may improve sleep.

❖ **Spiritual Reflection-** Be as informed and knowledgeable as possible. Utilize faith, belief systems, spiritual resources and support, if this is a part of your life.

❖ **Treasure memories-** Stories, experiences, words of wisdom, mannerisms, and such, are some of the best legacies that are gifted after a loss. Share these memories with family and friends, realizing that it is normal if you discover you laugh or cry. Consider memorializing your loss by planting a tree, donating time, services or funds to a special cause.

❖ **YOU are a unique individual-** No one grieves or copes in exactly the same way. Your experience will be influenced by a number of factors. Don't pressure or worry yourself by comparing your response to someone else's. Recovery occurs at your own individual pace.

Resources are available for you beyond your closest friends and family. If you feel you may benefit from some outside assistance, please call one of the numbers below, or seek other appropriate professional services.

Reactions to Crisis and Trauma

After a crisis or traumatic event (an event that causes unusually strong reactions and has the potential to overwhelm one's normal coping mechanism) it is common (and quite normal) for people to experience emotional aftershocks/stress reactions. Sometimes these occur immediately and sometimes it can be hours, days, weeks or months after the event. Reactions can last days, weeks and, in some cases even longer (depending on the impact/severity of the crisis or trauma). While it is impossible know exactly how an individual will react, it is important to understand that trauma affects people in many different ways. These reactions are part of the stress response and are not a sign of weakness or inability to do the job.

Having accurate information about typical reactions coupled with understanding & support from friends, co-workers, family or other loved ones can make big difference to people affected by traumatic events. Sometimes, however, that is not enough and professional assistance may be needed. This does not mean a person is weak, crazy, etc. It simply means that the event or combination of events was just too powerful or overwhelming for the person to manage alone.

Physical	Cognitive	Emotional	Relational	Behavioral	Spiritual
Flight, Fight or Freeze	Blaming	Anxiety	Withdrawal from family, coworkers, colleagues	Change in speech	Questions about faith
Shock, numbness	Confusion	Crying		Withdrawal	Run to or from God
Nausea	Poor attention	Guilt	Withdrawal from organizations or other affiliations	Emotional outbursts	Anger at God
Exhaustion	Poor decisions	Survivor guilt		Accident prone	Vulnerability and mortality
Muscle tremors, shakes or aches	Hard to concentrate	Numbing	Isolation	Potential for violence	Withdraw from faith and religion
Twitches	Memory problems	Grief	Stigma, racism, sexism, media response	Suspiciousness	Concern about hereafter
Chest pain	Hyper-vigilant	Disbelief		Loss/increase of appetite	
Fast pulse	Nightmares	Denial	Secondary injuries from friends, family, social & professional affiliations contribute to additional stress	Startle reaction	Questions about good and evil
Rapid heart rate	Intrusive images	Panic		Alcohol/drug consumption	Questioning God
Headaches	Poor problem solving	Startle response		Inability to rest	Redefining moral values
Weakness, fatigue	Difficulty calculating	Emotional shock		Pacing	Promising, bargaining & challenging God during times of duress or trauma
Dizziness	Difficulty identifying objects or people	Uncertainty	Unemployment or under-employment	Change in sexual function or sex drive	
Sweating	Difficulty remembering details	Depression like symptoms	Discontinued educational pursuits	Crying	Searching for meaning and hope
Elevated blood pressure	Time distortion	Apprehension	Lack of community or political involvement	Recklessness	
Chills	Auditory distortion	Irritability		Hyper-alert to environment	Concern about vengeance, justice and forgiveness
Trouble sleeping		Agitation		Ritualistic behavior	
Excessive sleeping		Anger		Criminal behavior	Spiritual "awakening"
Diarrhea		Outbursts		Loss of motivation	
Indigestion		Loss of emotional control		Excessive spending	
Non-specific body complaints		Euphoria			
		Obsessiveness			

Always seek medical help or additional assistance if there is even a question that it is needed!

~ This is a compilation of information inspired by the International Critical Incident Stress Foundation (ICISF) with contributions and input from a whole host of people dedicated to helping others.

THINGS TO TRY:

- **WITHIN THE FIRST 24 - 48 HOURS** periods of appropriate physical exercise, alternated with relaxation will alleviate some of the physical reactions.
- Structure your time; keep busy.
- You're normal and having normal reactions; don't label yourself crazy.
- Talk to people; talk is the most healing medicine.
- Be aware of numbing the pain with overuse of drugs or alcohol, you don't need to complicate this with a substance abuse problem.
- Reach out; people do care.
- Maintain as normal a schedule as possible.
- Spend time with others.
- Help your co-workers as much as possible by sharing feelings and checking out how they are doing.
- Give yourself permission to feel rotten and share your feelings with others.
- Keep a journal; write your way through those sleepless hours.
- Do things that feel good to you.
- Realize those around you are under stress.
- Don't make any big life changes.
- Do make as many daily decisions as possible restore a feeling of control over your life, i.e., if someone asks you what you want to eat, answer him even if you're not sure.
- Get plenty of rest.
- Don't try to fight reoccurring thoughts, dreams or flashbacks - they are normal and will decrease over time and become less painful.
- Eat well-balanced and regular meals (even if you don't feel like it).

FOR FAMILY MEMBERS & FRIENDS

- Listen carefully.
- Spend time with the traumatized person.
- Offer your assistance and a listening ear if (s)he has not asked for help.
- Reassure him that he is safe.
- Help him with everyday tasks like cleaning, cooking, caring for the family, minding children.
- Give him some private time.
- Don't take his anger or other feelings personally.
- Don't tell him that he is "lucky it wasn't worse;"

     ▲   A traumatized person is not consoled by those statements. Instead, tell him that you are sorry such an event has occurred and you want to understand and assist.

EXAMPLES OF ASSOCIATIVE/ENVIRONMENTAL (SENSORY TRIGGERS)

Smell of Nomex	Helicopters	Radio Traffic	Burning debris	Tree Branches
Thunderstorms	Aircraft	Air Tankers	Fire Alarms	Fuels/Smell:
Smoke	Chainsaws	Yelling/Loud Voices	Intense Heat	(Jet A, Saw Gas, Drip Mix)
Firelines	Pumps/Small Motors	Retardant/Foam	Any sensory input which was present at the time of the incident	

While many of these signs and signals are normal, seek immediate professional attention if they persist or become overwhelming!

Chapter Twenty-Three

References

Conn, Stephanie M. (2018) Increasing resiliency in police and emergency personnel. Routledge Publishing, New York, NY

Gilmartin, Kevin M. (2021). Emotional survival for law enforcement: A guide for officers and their families. E-S Press, Tucson, Az.

Stephens, Richard J. (2022) The calling: Seated at the table with the broken. Newman Springs Publishing, Red Bank, NJ.

Williams, Jason J. (2017) The need for law enforcement wellness interventions: a critical review. The sports journal. Retrieved on March 23, 2023, from https://thesportsjournal.org

Harper, Michael C. (2023). Enhancing Officer Safety and Survivability. International Association of Chief's of Police, Police Chief Magazine. Retrieved on 03/2/2023 from; https://www.policechiefmagazine.org/enhancing-officer-safety-survivability

Williams, Bradley (2018). The importance of exercise for stress management for police officers. Police Fit.com. Retrieved on 03/02/23 from https://www.policefit.com.au/blog/the-importance-of-exercise-for-stress-management-for-police-officers

Malmin, Mark, (2012) Changing Police Subculture. Retrieved from https://leb-fbi.gov/articles/featured-articles/changing-police-subculture. Retrieved on December 1, 2022.

Morin, Rich (2017). Police Culture. Pew Research center. Retrieved from https://www.pewresearch.org. Retrieved on January 13, 2023

Reed, Jon (2022) Writing and mental health: 8 psychological benefits of writing. Publishing talk. Retrieved from https://www.publishingtalk.org. Retrieved February 28, 2023.

Kirschmen, Ellen (2021) Cops and Shrink's: When to go to Therapy and Why. Psychology Today Magazine blog. Retrieved from https://www.psycologytoday.org.

Morgan, Amy (2021) 6 ways a peer support team has an officers back. Police 1. Retrieved from police1.com on January 4, 2023.

Conrad, Sean (2017). Protecting the protectors: the benefits of peer support groups in law enforcement. Leadership Command College. June 2017.

Afterword

Shadows

Richard J. Stephens Jr., MA

They whine, they cry, they expect me to care.

Their inconsideration for my time wears upon me like a monumental weight, destined to forever hold me against my will. Always bringing me strife, never allowing me rest; my existence seemingly is dependent upon their reach. I want to listen, I do feel, I have a heart but for now they must simply be strong as I am unable.

My mind is racing, thoughts wont cease, visions ascending, failing to decrease.

The Shadows are coming.

Shadows wearing the form of my thoughts and memories, better left forgotten. Closing mine eyes, surely, they will depart, forever to remain absent from afar. Dark shadows descending upon me as a thundering storm. Bent on destroying everything within its path, relentless and uncaring, hard yet unable to be restrained. My strength will conquer, surely it might, if not forever, just for tonight.

Dark shadows ascending as a sweltering wave, filling every crevice and void, remembering not my woes, caring little of my dismay, overtaking with rage, adding to my cage. Encircling my soul as a violent wind, dark and powerful, consuming all that is good and useful, distorting the very structure of my existence. Smiling and screaming as it overtakes me. Struggling to breath, I sink deeper, treading for life, yet I find no footing. Growing ever closer to the abyss of my destruction, void of warmth, I am cold, so very cold. This is my destiny, overtaken by memories, crushed by thoughts, restrained and unmovable. Fearing no man yet fearing myself for the shadows have consumed all life in itself.

What, upon my eyes do I see? through the clouds, drawing ever closer...a ray, a tiny ray, glimmering light splitting the darkness.

I reach for the warmth, but the shadows draw my hand, dragging me back, further into the deep, deep sand, far from the approaching safety, restraining me, binding me, preventing me. Battling the warmth, the shadows stir as a monumental captor refusing to surrender the ground they have conquered. Upon my eyes the light grows brighter, bight as an emboldened protector, chasing the fleeing darkness upon its retreat, Voices emboldened as heroes upon the horizon, breaking the grasp of the shadows of the mind, torment running, ease prevails through the consuming shield of hope which is unveiled.

Focus is regained, gazing upon the form of a friend, a voice through the darkness, the light now ascends.

May I never grow weary of lending the hand, never fearing unleashing the light for a friend. The time, which was taken to fight off the dark, brings forth hope that one day my shadows will depart.

www.ingramcontent.com/pod-product-compliance
Lightning Source LLC
Chambersburg PA
CBHW060243030426
42335CB00014B/1580